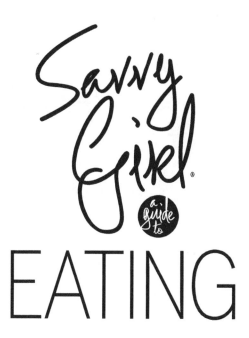

EATING

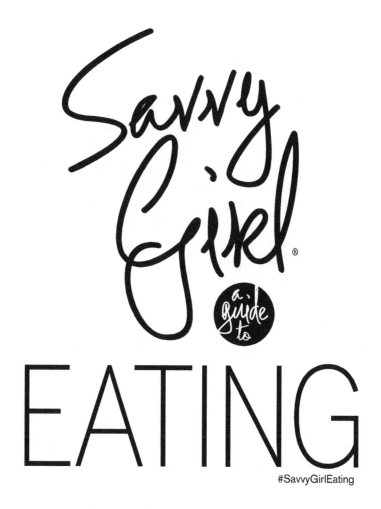

EATING

#SavvyGirlEating

SAVVY GIRL, BRITTANY DEAL *and*
SUMNER BROOKS MPH, RDN, CSSD
FOUNDER OF NOT ON A DIET

Savvy Girl: A Guide to Eating
Brittany Deal, Sumner Brooks
Copyright © 2014 by Brittany Deal
All Rights Reserved

Content Editor: Meghan Rabbitt
Copyeditor: Rachelle Mandik
Cover & Interior Design: Tara Long/Dotted Line Design, LLC

Ordering Information:
Orders by US trade bookstores and wholesalers.
Please e-mail Savvy Girl at hello@savvygirl.net

Published in the United States of America
ISBN 978-0-9897109-4-7
First Edition

PHOTO CREDITS: *Cover* © GettyImages/ManuWe
Interior p. 9 ©Karramba Production; p. 12 ©Bildagentur Zoonar GmbH; p. 15 ©Deymos.HR; p. 22 ©Diana Taliun; p. 22 ©antpkr; p. 25 ©lanych; p. 25 ©Preto Perola; p. 27 ©bikeriderlondon; p. 32 ©jajaladdawan; p. 39 ©istockphoto/ WeeraDanwilai; p. 42 ©irin-k; p. 45 ©Jill Chen; p. 50 ©Ostancov Vladislav; p. 56 ©istockphoto/JulNichols; p.58 ©istockphoto/ TaphouseStudios; p. 70 ©Africa Studio; p. 70 ©istockphoto/robynmac; p.71 ©istockphoto/kickimages; p. 74 ©Filip Krstic; p. 78 ©Kim Reinick; p. 83 ©iko; p. 86 ©istockphoto/ Givaga; p.93 ©istockphoto/ DMP1; p.94 ©istockphoto/ gbh007; p.97 ©Stephen Mcsweeny; p. 99 ©David Guyler; p. 104 ©istockphoto/DebbiSmirnoff; p. 107 ©Gianna Stadelmyer; p. 109 ©trucic; p. 110 ©LoveFreedom; p. 111 ©Sofiaworld.

Meet the Authors

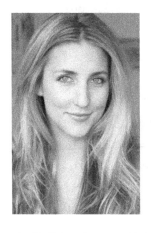

MEET BRITTANY

Brittany Deal is the founder and CEO of Savvy Girl, a lifestyle brand that publishes micro how-to books that help women thrive. As a lifetime lover of learning, Brittany craved the knowledge nonfiction books promised to offer, but found most of them painfully boring to read. After giving up on another how-to book in the middle of a quarter-life crisis trip to the Bolivian Amazon, Brittany had an epiphany: We are drowning in information yet starved for knowledge. With the idea of creating one go-to source for information-rich, yet concise books written in a "girlfriend-to-girlfriend" style, Brittany launched Savvy Girl. Brittany partners with top-notch experts to co-create these informative, fun, and quick reads so women can get savvy— and then get back to living their fabulous lives.

FOLLOW BRITTANY

@BrittanyDeal
@BrittanyDeal
BrittanyDeal.com

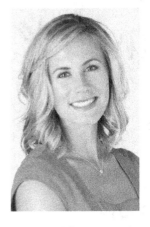

MEET SUMNER BROOKS, MPH, RDN, CSSD

Sumner Brooks is the founder of *Not On A Diet*, a private nutrition therapy practice in Los Angeles, where she helps her clients become "Intuitive Eaters"—a nutrition philosophy that encourages people to ditch diets for good and listen to what their bodies want. Brooks has extensive experience and training: She's a registered dietitian nutritionist, board-certified sports specialty dietitian, a certified Intuitive Eating counselor, and received her master's of public health (MPH) from UCLA. Thanks to this extensive education and experience, Sumner mixes science and self-compassion to help others achieve ultimate wellness. Her success in the field of nutrition counseling is due in large part to Sumner's own past confusion about food and heartache from disordered eating. She understands these are debilitating issues facing so many, and her passion for preventing and treating eating issues inspires her daily work with clients, as well as her writing, community activism, and public speaking.

FOLLOW SUMNER
@MyDietitian
@IntuitiveEatingRD
NotOnADiet.com

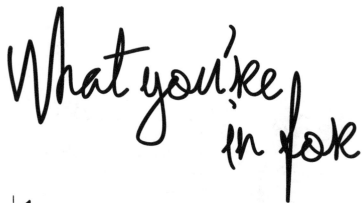
What you're in for

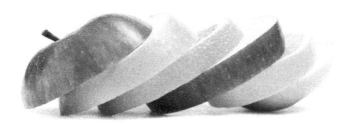

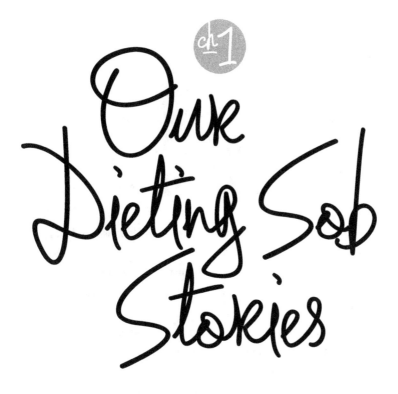

Our Dieting Sob Stories

BRITTANY'S STORY

[**BRITT:** It was New Year's Day morning and the throbbing pain of a hangover from a New Year's Eve wedding had me out of bed at an early hour. Memories of dancing the night away, bottomless Champagne, and lots of glitter and confetti (some of which was still stuck to me) meant I succeeded in ending 2012 with a bang. With a freshly brewed cup of coffee in one hand and a notepad and pen in the other I was ready to charge into 2013 with some New Year's resolutions.

I've always loved resolutions because I love the idea of starting fresh. But this year's New Year's resolutions weren't making me feel as invigorated as usual. I scanned my list and realized why: my resolution to "lose weight." That darn resolution had been on my list every single year. No matter

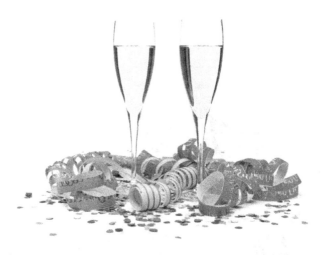

how hard I tried, I just couldn't seem to cross it off my list, and it was officially starting to irk me.

So I pulled out my pen again. Next to my weight-loss goal, I wrote "for good" with an underline and far too many exclamation marks.

For most of my twenties, I tried every workout routine imaginable to get "skinny." I joined (and quit) about three different gyms, I took Pilates classes at $25 a pop, I forced myself to go to six a.m. boot camps, and I pushed myself to nearly fainting levels at circuit-training classes. I began each new workout regimen thinking it would be my golden ticket to "skinny bitch" land.

After years of intense, hour-long workouts I finally had an epiphany: It must be the food I eat that's preventing me from reaching my ideal weight. So I started dieting. Whether it was a juice cleanse, no-carb plan, or becoming vegetarian, I was game for any and all restrictive eating plans that promised to help me drop pounds.

Nothing worked.

One Thanksgiving, the holiday of no-holds-barred gluttony, I found myself extra-focused on dieting. Out of determination and self-loathing, I made a crazy plan for myself: I would work out twice a day, count calories, and cut back my sugar and alcohol intake significantly. After three months of torture, I weighed less, but food had become the enemy.

Like with all diets, I eventually couldn't sustain this way-too-restrictive plan. I dreaded my workouts and deeply missed my favorite foods. When I ditched my crazy diet and started eating my favorite foods again (hello, pizza!), I would often eat more than I needed because I was worried that I'd start another diet and officially never see pizza again. Eventually, the weight I'd lost came back—along with the old feelings of defeat and a worse-than-ever body image.

So, on New Year's Day 2013, I felt a renewed sense of hope when I made that promise to myself to figure out the weight-loss thing for good. To make sure it was for good, I decided to work with a dietitian. Now, this might sound like a healthy move—but dieting had screwed up how I thought about food. Case in point: my goal was to hire a dietitian who, I had hoped, would tell me that if I didn't eat "clean" or "raw" or "vegan" every day, I would never reach my ideal weight. I thought that if she could just scare me into being "good," I would be able to eat the "right" foods and finally get skinny and stay skinny.

Luckily, I didn't find the dietitian I was looking for. Instead, I found nutrition therapist Sumner Brooks.

Sumner taught me that the key to being healthy and feeling great in my body is through a non-dieting approach to eating. Turns out that while not being on a diet was the exact opposite of what I was looking for, it was exactly what I needed. What Sumner taught me transformed my life and my health and finally made it so that "lose weight" hasn't made an appearance on my New Year's resolutions lists since. And I'm pretty confident that phrase will stay off my resolutions lists for good. Before we dive into exactly why diets don't work, I want you to first hear how Sumner's own dieting story led her to become a dietitian, and how her experience has helped her coach people on how to fix their relationship with food, be comfortable in their bodies, and kiss dieting good-bye.]

SUMNER'S STORY

I approached the glass doors of Cold Stone Creamery feeling both anxiety and excitement. I looked up and down the street to make sure no one I knew was nearby. Once I was in the clear, I walked inside and indulged in the scent of sweet vanilla and freshly baked waffle cones. I could order anything my little heart desired.

I had spent the weekend nearly starving myself because my overly critical boyfriend had been visiting from out of town. He wasn't shy about letting me know that he'd noticed the ten pounds I'd put on since we met. I was dieting to please him—and, well, to please everyone in my life (or that's what I thought, anyway). I constantly believed that I would be more accepted, more valued, and more worthy if I could control my weight and body. But after I dropped him off at the San Diego Airport, I couldn't wait to finally eat.

Once I'd stuffed myself with ice cream, a familiar wave of guilt and shame rolled in. I was a twenty-three-year-old nutrition student, vice president of the San Diego State University Student Nutrition Organization, and I had recently been accepted into one of the most competitive dietetic internship programs in the state. ..

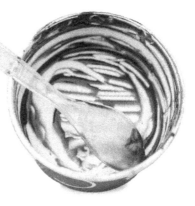

...and there I was, shamefully and secretly eating ice cream.

HOW I GOT THEI_

Dieting and food was running my life, to the point that I felt like a prisoner in my own mind and body. From the moment I woke up, I analyzed my body for signs of improvement or proof of the damage I'd done the day before. Then, the onslaught of questions would hit: Had I worked out enough this week? Had I earned a day off from the gym? What was I allowed to eat today?

If I felt thin, life was good. If I felt fat, I was depressed, moody, and irritable. I ached for ways to escape this mental prison and often used alcohol to quiet my own self-criticism.

Friends would tease me for being the "healthy" one, the "good" one, and for always going to the gym even the day after a late night out. What they never knew and didn't understand was that it didn't feel like a choice to me; I was just paying the penance for indulging the night before.

You see, no one ever talks about how bad it feels to always be on a diet. The only time anyone is ever bragging about their diet is at the start, when the pride of sticking to it for a few days is highest or when they've seen some initial weight loss. No one gushes about the diet they didn't stay on or the plan that worked at first and then made them gain all of that weight back (and then some) when they fell off the wagon. No one brags about how bad it feels to wake up and begin the cycle of body shame and judgment day after day.

As a nutrition student, I had all the information I needed on how to be healthy—yet I was more interested in knowing what I needed to eat and do to be thin. The harder I tried to be a perfect eater, the more I felt cravings and the urge to binge. The more pressure I put on myself to be skinny, the more my body wavered back and forth, like a pendulum, between overfed and starved. Of course, dieting never helped anything fall into place.

MY "AHA" MOMENT

After years of waking up every morning criminalizing myself for something I ate the day before, or for feeling too fat in my clothes, or for having too much cellulite and a too-soft belly, I woke up one morning and did something different.

My normal morning routine was to have a cup of coffee, exercise to burn as many calories as I could manage, and then eat a light, low-carb breakfast. Then by midday I'd be back at the fridge and telling myself that I had no willpower. But my aha moment happened when I thought to myself, You don't have to lose weight today. Why don't you just see what it feels like to eat for your hunger instead of eating to change your body? Afterward I felt an immediate sense of relief.

This change in thought pattern came from reading the book Intuitive Eating by Evelyn Tribole and Elyse Resch. Maybe, I thought, my body isn't so terrible after all. I was surprised at how much I enjoyed that breakfast, carbs and all, in an entirely new way, and I also remember how my mood, my energy, and my outlook on life was different in a way I didn't know how to explain. No matter where you're at with your physical size or shape, finding a way to accept your here-and-now body and to let go of the shame and guilt you have about eating is the doorway to moving from the detrimental dieting cycle to a place of freedom and peace with food and your body.

After discovering the "non-dieting" approach to eating I started to see changes for the better. I learned that dieting itself was actually the root problem of all of my eating issues, and within a few weeks of learning how to implement a non-dieting approach, I felt more comfortable, healthy, and in control than I had in years. From there, I reached out for support, changed the way I taught nutrition (this was huge for me, as a lot of my healing came from helping others do the same), and kissed dieting good-bye for good.

Since my own transformation from an unhappy, unhealthy dieter to a happy and healthy non-dieter, I've been on a mission to help free people from the dieting cycle that keeps them in their own food prisons. There is solid research backing up the fact that dieting leads to disordered eating, weight gain, and clinical eating disorders. What I now know for sure is that it's impossible to realize how much dieting holds you back until you are finally freed from trying to control every bite.

Next Up

➔ How the dieting cycle keeps you sucked in

➔ How chronic dieting can harm your body

➔ Why a non-dieting approach to eating works

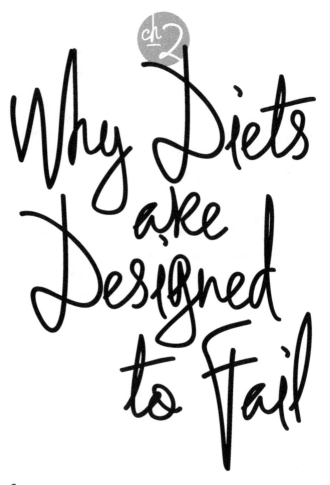

Why Diets are Designed to Fail

[BRITT: How many diets do you think you've tried in your life? More than you can count, right? And how many magazines have you reached for because one of the headlines read, CELEBRITY X DROPPED 20LBS! STEAL HER SECRETS! As if the Holy Grail to a great bum, thin thighs, and no cellulite is waiting for us on page 62 of a $2.99 magazine.

Deep down, we're smarter than that. We all know that those headlines are designed to sell magazines and that next week's headline will rave about a totally different diet. But these magazines and dieting books have marketing ninjas behind them who know that you and I can't help but peek inside—you know, just in case the secret to a perfect body really is on page 62.

There's a saying that goes "The definition of insanity is doing the same thing over and over again and expecting a different result." Based on those wise words, you'd think we'd all realize by now that we are insane to keep dieting. But I will cut us all some slack here because this saying is so old that you can bet the originator wasn't staring at a gorgeous bikini-clad-celebrity on the cover of US Weekly every time he checked out at the grocery store.

Dieting, on the surface, also seems like it should work. The whole "eat healthy, cut back on calories, and the weight will come off" seems like a simple enough equation, right? But what's missing is the mental torment that diets cause, which inevitably results in feelings of failure.

This is where our non-dieting guru, Sumner, helps set us straight. She'll explain exactly why diets are designed to fail and why the failure of one diet spurs the search for the next one, thus keeping us in the "dieting cycle." Once you understand what's really going on below the surface, you won't be lured by those headlines and you won't be tempted to repeat the same destined-to-fail dieting cycle over and over again. Sanity restored after reading one short chapter? I promise!]

Brittany is right: Diets have mad sex appeal. They tempt us with their promise that if we follow specific advice, we will lose weight and our life will finally be catapulted to new levels of success. We believe that if we can just achieve our ideal weight, perfection on all fronts will follow.

The truth is, you're likely reading this right now because diets never made anything better at all. In fact, they've probably made your life worse, or at the very least more complicated.

Ultimately, diets fail because they trigger feelings of food insecurity, cravings, rebellion, and food obsession. The dieting cycle is a trap because the inevitable failure of one diet results in feelings of depression, guilt, and shame. And so the start of the next diet begins with even more vengeance.

THE DIETING CYCLE

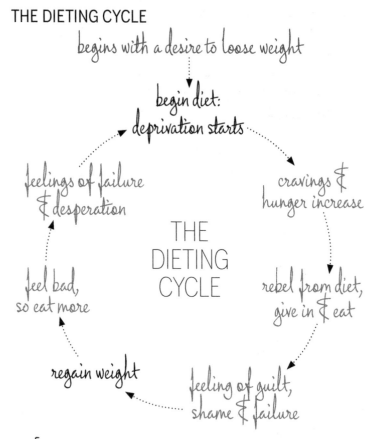

begins with a desire to loose weight

begin diet:
deprivation starts

feelings of failure
& desperation

cravings &
hunger increase

THE
DIETING
CYCLE

feel bad,
so eat more

rebel from diet,
give in & eat

regain weight

feeling of guilt,
shame & failure

[BRITT: It's starting to make sense why dieting is a billion-dollar industry, right? As soon as your last diet fails, the next expert with their method to "blast your fat away in twenty-one days" is ready to take your money and get you back on track to your next dieting failure.]

Dieting, after a while, can happen even when you don't think you're on a diet. That's why we refer to it as the "dieting mentality." It can be very automatic and even subconscious for an experienced dieter. Counting points; following food rules; adding up calories, carbs, and fat grams—it's all part of dieting.

DIETING IS LIKE BEING IN FOOD JAIL:
Our desire to lose weight puts us there, and the prison guards—Guilt and Shame—keep us locked up. With each diet, your ability to decide what and how much you want to eat is stripped away from you a little more until you've completely forgotten what it's like to eat without guilt.

YOUR BODY VS. A DIET: WHY IT'S NOT A FAIR FIGHT

It's amazing how our bodies are able to control and maintain weight on their own. When the body detects that it is not getting enough calories, nutrients, or carbohydrates, chemicals in the brain—along with the hunger hormone, ghrelin—kick into gear, making us think about food and crave more of it while gradually slowing down the metabolism to conserve energy.

Diet Buzzword

GHRELIN: A hormone produced naturally by the body to regulate appetite control and tell you when it's time to eat.

Ghrelin actually makes high-calorie foods look more appetizing and low-calorie foods less appealing—hence why that chocolate molten-lava cake looks so much more appealing than the fruit bowl. Why does this sneaky little hormone do this? Because ghrelin's purpose is to make sure you're eating enough. The trick with ghrelin is that you have to eat enough calories and nutrients for this hunger hormone to subside. So, if you eat a huge bowl of cucumbers or rice cakes, your body will still know it hasn't had enough nutrition and ghrelin will stay elevated until you finally give your body what it needs.

This is why overeating as a response to undereating is not only normal, it's predictable. Willpower has nothing to do with this. Your brain is always going to win; after all, its job is to make sure you survive.

So, when ghrelin, along with your body's other natural hunger mechanisms, is making a lot of noise but you're trying to ignore it because you're on a diet, you subconsciously begin to feel aggravated that you're not "allowed" to have what you want and need. Your aggravation and deprivation turns into rebellion, and the moment you take even just one bite of non-diet-approved food (which, by the way, you desperately need at this point) you feel you've failed, there's no turning back, and you eat anything and everything you crave—usually the forbidden foods you've been avoiding while dieting.

[BRITT: What you should be hearing right now is that when you eat five stalks of celery for lunch and then plow through a box of crackers before dinner, it's not a sign that you have no willpower. It's a biological response that is designed to keep you alive and kickin'. Your body doesn't know that your calorie restriction is self-imposed.]

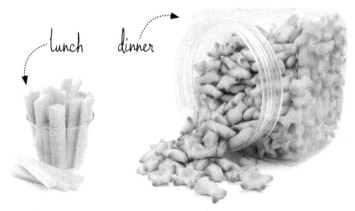

lunch   dinner

22

HOW CHRONIC DIETING CAN HARM YOUR BODY

Did you know that chronic dieting can change your body composition? When you lose weight quickly by following a low-calorie diet, your body is still going to keep working and burning the necessary energy required to keep your body functioning as usual. If you're not eating enough calories, guess where that energy is going to come from? Your muscle tissue.

While you might be thinking, Great, my thigh muscles have some room to give, your body doesn't spot-treat. Muscle breakdown happens all over, including the muscles that are your vital organs. Your heart, brain, and other organs can become weak when this muscle loss occurs, and they'll even fail as a result of chronic food restriction. And here's the real kicker: as your body loses muscle, it holds on to fat, increasing your body's fat percentage. This is one of the most frustrating aspects for chronic dieters who can't understand why their "healthy eating" isn't giving them the bikini body of their dreams.

The good news? When you return to a consistent way of eating that adequately feeds your body, you can regain your muscle and nudge your metabolism back to a revved-up rate.

HAVE YOU BEEN BRAINWASHED BY DIETS?

When we start a new diet, we do so from a desire to get control over our health and the way we look. However, a dieting mentality only gives us the illusion that we are in control.

I have sat through hundreds of initial consultations with clients who have been chronic dieters, and sadly, what I hear tends to be a lot of the same thing:

▸ "I try so hard, and I just can't control myself."

▸ "I just need more willpower and I need you to help me stay accountable."

- "I'm really good all day—and then when I get home from work I'm out of control."

- "I was so bad last night because I knew I was starting this program today. I went to bed feeling terrible and guilty after a big pizza and too much ice cream."

Guilt. Shame. Self-loathing. Anger. Sadness. Hopelessness. Failure. Unworthiness.

Hardly the feelings one expects to have when the goal is to feel in control. Instead, these are the feelings that overcome us when we "cheat" on a diet—the feelings that prompt us to start the next restrictive eating plan. The dieting mentality brainwashes us into thinking that we are the problem.

What all of my chronic dieters who've turned into happy, healthy, non-dieters didn't realize in the beginning is that all of these plans and shakes and pills were not designed to work. Most of these diets are trying to turn a profit from your desperation to lose weight. In fact, the vast majority of diets are not based on science. That's why we call them "fads." While some diets sound more sensible than others, almost all of them still require you to follow food rules and deprive yourself. And, as you've likely experienced, it's that deprivation that'll prompt you to rebel sooner or later.

[BRITT: I felt so relieved when Sumner told me that I was doing nothing wrong and that my overeating was related to how dieting was affecting my mind and body, not that I had no willpower. This made me see everything differently. Suddenly, I was no longer the problem—the diets were the problem.]

Diets cause another unhealthy behavior as well. Think about what percentage of your day you spend thinking about food, weight, or dieting. Right now, grab a pen and start tallying up the number of times a day—and the minutes you spend each time—thinking about food, obsessing about your body, and pep-talking (or shaming) yourself about what you should or shouldn't be eating.

Does the number surprise you?

If you're spending that much time worrying and obsessing over what to eat, feeling guilty after a binge, or overexercising to "make up for" the dessert you had last night, what else in your life might you be missing out on? How much more fun could you be having if you spent this time and brainpower on yourself, your career, or your relationships?

Once you stop dieting and let your body tell you when, what, and how much to eat, you'll be amazed at what you can accomplish and how free you'll feel. What if the next time you ate a slice of pizza it had the same emotional impact as if you'd eaten an apple?

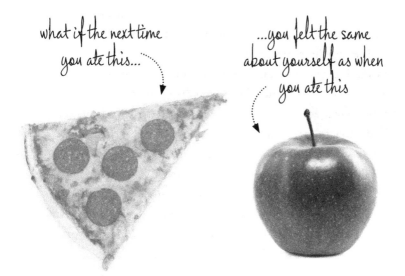

what if the next time you ate this...

...you felt the same about yourself as when you ate this

It may sound too good to be true, but ask any non-dieter and they'll tell you this kind of thinking is possible. It's how we're designed to interact with food from the moment we're born. Infants and children know when to eat and when to stop eating. It's when we let food rules, restrictions, and statements that start with "I should" get in the way of the body's hunger signals that food becomes a problem.

If you can commit your energy to learning to listen to your body and develop a new relationship with food, I promise that you will be the absolute best version of your healthy self. It happened to me. I see it happen to my clients. And it can happen to you, too.

"BUT I STILL JUST WANT TO LOSE WEIGHT!"

I know, I know—you want to lose weight. Or at least that's what you think you want. When society constantly reinforces that (1), you can never be too skinny and (2), the only way to lose weight is to restrict and avoid anything high in calories, it makes this mental shift a bit scary. I get that.

Although you may feel like you're not in your healthiest body right now, if you keep attempting to fix that with more diets, you'll get nowhere. Sometimes this starts with an adjustment in expectations about weight loss. For example, just because that bout of mono you had in college meant you got down to your lowest weight ever, that doesn't mean that it's an achievable, healthy weight for you now.

Also, weight does not determine a person's health risk—behaviors do. People can be healthy at a range of sizes, but being thin does not equal being healthy. If you are not already within your genetically designed healthy weight range, which is different for everyone, losing weight may feel more comfortable for you. But you have to let your body naturally and gradually lose extra weight as a result of changing your thought patterns around food—not by forever swearing off bagels and birthday cake.

So, are you ready to break free of the never-ending dieting cycle and let yourself out of food prison? Are you ready for a better way of living?

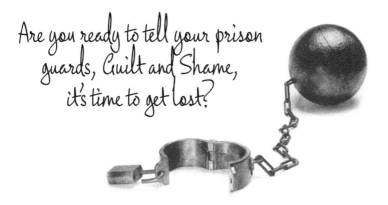

Are you ready to tell your prison guards, Guilt and Shame, it's time to get lost?

WHY NOT DIETING WILL WORK FOR YOU—FOR GOOD

Ditching diets doesn't mean eating crap all the time, stuffing your face and not caring, and gaining weight as a result. It means caring even more about your body and your health. By taking on a non-dieting mentality and learning to listen to and trust your body, you'll naturally settle at a weight that is healthy for you over time.

I know that sounds dangerous. You're thinking, Trust . . . myself? But I will only eat "bad" food if I listen to myself!

Trust me on this one, you won't only eat "bad" food. You will learn to trust yourself around food and, over time, you will choose the foods that make you feel good. Without dieting, there is no deprivation, no crazy ghrelin overload, no reason to rebel against those self-imposed rules and eat more than you need. That's because no one—and I mean no one—can ever deprive you from the right amount of food that you need.

What we're going to teach you in this book involves three main concepts:

1 Finding satisfaction by listening to your body

2 Letting go of emotional and mindless eating

3 Achieving body acceptance and great self-care

Keep in mind that shifting from a dieter to a Savvy Eater is a process. It will take time, and you're going to need to have some patience with yourself as you go. Congratulations, girl. You are now on your way to freeing yourself from the dieting cycle and feeling your best ever!

NOTE TO READER:

In this book I occasionally refer to non-dieters and Savvy Eaters as Intuitive Eaters, based on the well-researched eating model known as Intuitive Eating. Intuitive Eating was first developed in the 1990s by two revolutionary and savvy registered dietitians—Elyse Resch, MS, RDN, and Evelyn Tribole, MS, RDN—who realized that putting clients on calorie-restricted diet plans was not going to make them healthier or help them form a healthy relationship with food. Intuitive Eating is now a widely practiced approach used by professionals in the fields of eating psychology and nutrition all over the world, and has been helping people become healthier and happier eaters for more than twenty years.

[BRITT: When I first started working with Sumner I didn't even realize how dieting had brainwashed me. Learning to be a Savvy Eater finally freed me from food prison and from all of the negative thoughts that kept me locked up. I had no idea how much dieting had affected other areas of my life until I got out of the cycle. I only wish I would have discovered this approach sooner.

Here is a diagram that shows what my life was like before and after becoming a Savvy Eater.]

My Life as a Dieter

- ○ Obsessed with food and being a "perfect" eater

- ○ Always trying to count calories and lose weight

- ○ Always feeling guilty for eating anything that wasn't kale

- ○ Hating myself for lacking the willpower to avoid my forbidden foods.

- ○ Approaching food like it was all-or-nothing

- ○ Not trusting myself around food

- ○ Fearing going out to eat

- ○ Having a terrible body image

- ○ Dreading working out

- ○ Being unaware of my emotional eating habits

Now as a Savvy Eater

- ○ Never counting calories or worrying about food

- ○ Eating the foods I like and not depriving myself

- ○ Never feeling guilty after I eat

- ○ Not trying to make up for past meals that felt uncomfortable

- ○ Avoiding all-or-nothing thinking about food

- ○ Loving going out to eat

- ○ Feeling totally in control around food

- ○ Loving my body

- ○ Getting active in ways that feel good to me

- ○ Learning alternative ways to soothe myself and deal with my emotions instead of using food

Next Up

 Why an all-or-nothing approach to eating doesn't work

 How to eat without feeling guilty

 Is aiming for moderation the goal?

ch 3

Don't cut
the Pasta
Cut the
Don'ts,
Shoulds,
and Can'ts

[BRITT: A few years ago I was on my way to an Italian restaurant for a friend's birthday dinner. As I drove to the party, I set an intention to avoid the pasta dishes and have only one bite of birthday cake. I had worked so hard all week to eat "clean" and hit the gym every day. I didn't want to let one night out ruin my efforts.

When we sat down, the server delivered a basket of piping-hot bread with garlic-infused dipping oil. My friends lunged for

It took every ounce of willpower in me to decline paradise in carbohydrate form.

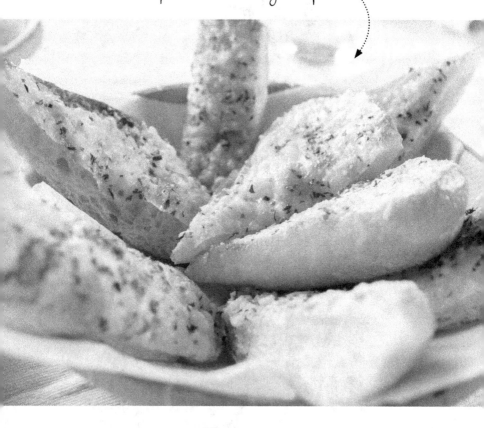

it and practically moaned in unison after their first bites. Then, as my friends ordered gnocchi and fettuccine, I asked for the chopped veggie salad. Dressing on the side, of course.

It felt like a lifetime waiting for our dinners to arrive, and minute by minute, the scent of garlicky oil and freshly baked bread taunted me. I hadn't eaten a carb all week and as my agitation grew, the hungry girl inside me got louder and louder. "Dooooo it." she whispered. I caved and inhaled what was left of the bread.

I felt guilty immediately, so I justified my actions by making another rule: "This slip-up will be OK as long as you eat only half of your salad." When my plain salad arrived and half of it was forbidden, I felt extra-deprived. I couldn't help but look around and feel envious of all the creamy, fragrant pasta dishes sitting in front of everyone else. How can they order those meals? I thought to myself. These dishes must be over 1,000 calories per plate. Don't they know how many calories they've just wasted?

A rebellious storm began brewing in my mind, fueled by feelings of guilt and deprivation. The next thing I knew I was reaching for more bread, more oil, and by the end of the meal I had practically licked my salad bowl clean and could already taste that birthday cake. Sure enough, I ate every last bite of that, too.

When I got home, I started planning my double workout penance for Saturday morning and vowed to start fresh the next day. "I'll try harder tomorrow," I vowed, "and I will really cut carbs once and for all."]

Dieters like Brittany try so hard to restrict certain foods because they want to lose weight, eat right, and be healthy. However, dieting has the opposite effect. In the Italian restaurant, Brittany's self-imposed food rules caused her to feel deprived—

and to rebel as a result. The catch is that if Brittany had gone into this dinner with full permission to eat what she was craving, she wouldn't have had any reason to rebel. She would have left feeling more comfortably full and satiated, and she probably would've even consumed fewer total calories. Even better, she would've skipped the emotional roller coaster of self-abuse.

At first it may be difficult to believe that when you give yourself permission to eat what you want, the urge to rebel and to overeat gradually goes away. But eventually you will learn what it feels like to eat to feel satisfied. Don't underestimate yourself.

HOW TO CUT THE DON'TS, SHOULDS, AND CAN'TS

Think about how often you tell yourself you "shouldn't" or you "can't" have a particular food because you think it's bad for you. Then ask yourself, "How has this worked for me?"

First off, let's recognize that most, if not all, of the food and dieting don'ts, shoulds, and can'ts you've been trying to adhere to represent a type of thinking we call all-or-nothing. You either can or you can't, and there's no in between. Getting out of this all-or-nothing thinking is where true change begins: It's time to recognize—and embrace—that you can be healthy and eat a variety of foods. (Yes, even foods like pasta, dessert, and pizza.)

The secret to making this change in how you think about food comes in two steps:

① *Break the rules.*

② *Ditch the guilt.*

FIRST UP, HERE'S HOW TO BE A RULE-BREAKER . . .

IGNORE YOUR OLD DIET "SHOULDS"

Any self-talk or food rules that start with "I can't have that" or "I shouldn't order that" are all dieting thoughts that will prevent you from being a Savvy Eater. When you hear thoughts about what your body "should" look like or what you "should" weigh, remember that no one—not even a doctor or an expert—really knows what you "should" weigh or eat. That is up to your genetic makeup.

We know for a fact that people can be healthy at a range of sizes and weights, and it's important for you to connect with what healthy means to you. If there were no scales, how would you define what healthy is for your body? You are the expert when it comes to what works and feels good for you, so ultimately you will rebel against anyone who tries to tell you what to eat or what not to eat. Pressure to reach a certain weight will keep you from giving yourself permission to eat what you crave.

FORGET "GOOD VS. BAD" THINKING

As a child, you didn't see a bagel and say to yourself, "Bad carbs!" or look at a cupcake and say, "Fat bomb!" Over the years, you've been taught certain rules by the media, our culture, and probably even your friends and family members who pit "good" foods (fruits and veggies and other health-promoting foods) against "bad" ones (sugar-filled desserts, fats, and breads). Odds are you've been following these food rules with the belief that if you chose only foods from the "good" list, you will lose weight.

So, how has that worked out for you?

I'm going to take a wild guess here and say there's a good chance it's turned you into a little food rebel, waiting for opportunities to indulge in off-limits foods.

As much as these diets made you believe "bad" foods are the enemy, the reality is eating more food than your body needs is what leads to weight gain, and there is no certain food or food group to blame. The point here is that you don't have to keep feeding yourself only veggies and egg whites; you can eat yummy foods and still be healthy and look and feel your best.

NEWS FLASH:
You can gain weight by eating more than you need of any food, whether it's orange slices or Thin Mints. What it comes down to is listening to your body and the signals it gives you about how much food you need. Nutritious foods are essential for health, but not having a healthy relationship with food can lead to the overeating that's causing you so much pain.

GIVE YOURSELF PERMISSION TO EAT WHAT YOU WANT

Decide that you will start allowing yourself to eat what you want in the moment. Now, this doesn't mean you need to make a beeline for the grocery store to fill up on all the yummy foods you haven't been eating. Instead, make a list of the foods you know you love, but that you don't allow yourself to have. Once you have that list, think about which, if any, of those foods you want to start eating again. Giving yourself permission to eat without feeling bad about it makes all foods emotionally equal. Instead of hearing the guilty thoughts, enjoy the food and sense when you've had enough.

Case in point: I've had numerous clients who've struggled with fro-yo binges. Fat-free and low-carb frozen yogurt is oftentimes one of the only ice cream–like foods dieting rules allow. However, one bite of any sweet, frozen dessert is going to create urges to overeat in order to make up for prior deprivation. When these clients allow themselves to have a frozen dessert as often as they want, their urges to binge gradually melt away.

Giving yourself permission to eat what you want, when you want it, means proving to yourself that you are allowed to eat the foods you crave without feeling guilty. When you're eating, remind yourself that if you want more tomorrow, you can have more, so you can stop at a place that leaves you feeling pleasantly full rather than sickly stuffed. Even just knowing that you don't have to deprive yourself can ease the tension and anxiety surrounding your food choices and reduce your urge to eat more than you really need.

BRITT: SO I HAVE PERMISSION TO EAT, BUT IT'S ALL ABOUT MODERATION, RIGHT?

SUMNER: Not exactly. Even though moderation is a very common dieting tip, there's no need to decide how much you should eat before you actually start eating. Starting your meal with a predetermined limit creates a feeling of perceived deprivation, and you may be tempted to rebel as a result. (Remember what happened when Brittany told herself she could have just one bite of birthday cake?) How can you really know ahead of time how much food it will take for you to feel satisfied, anyway? You can't. Sometimes that may mean having more than the "one serving" amount listed on a food label, or it may mean having less. Your goal is to learn to trust yourself by giving yourself full permission to eat what you need to feel satisfied.

To start breaking the food "rules," you need to train your brain to have different thought patterns. And the good news here is that there is scientific proof that you can do this: It's called neuroplasticity. Neuroplasticity is the brain's ability to reorganize itself by forming new neural connections. Practice an alternative way of thinking and behaving, and you can create new habits. Not sure where to start? Here are some examples of how to swap your old "dieting mentality" for a new, savvier way of thinking:

DITCH THIS SHOULD: "I should order the lowest-calorie option on the menu."

GET SAVVY: "I have permission to order what sounds the most satisfying to me."

DITCH THIS CAN'T: "I can't eat that cupcake. I'll gain weight."

GET SAVVY: "If I allow myself to eat that cupcake, I don't know how much of it I'll actually want to eat. Even just a couple bites may satisfy my craving for something sweet. I'm allowed to have as much as feels right to me."

DITCH THIS SHOULD: "I should eat light next week because I didn't count calories all weekend, and now I'm sure I've gained five pounds."

GET SAVVY: "I feel like I may have eaten more than I needed this weekend, so what can I learn from how it felt to eat that way? Why did I feel the need to do that? What would I like to do differently that will feel better next time?"

DITCH THIS DON'T: "I don't eat processed foods because they're unhealthy and will make me gain weight."

GET SAVVY: "Extreme thinking about food never works. All foods can fit within a healthy diet."

NEXT, HERE'S HOW TO DITCH THE GUILT . . .
STOP THINKING THAT GUILT IS HELPING YOU

Most dieters believe guilt is what helps them get back on track the next day. What you may not realize is that guilt, which sets in while you're eating or even before you start eating, is often what causes you to eat more than you need or eat impulsively because of the last-supper mentality. (You know, the "This is the last time, I swear!" mantra you put on repeat when you're about to dig in to a forbidden food.)

However, the truth is that I've seen hundreds of women let go of guilt, and it has never caused them to eat wildly out of control.

You may be cautiously afraid to let go of guilt, but the sooner you can accept it's not doing anything for you, the sooner you'll be able to find a way of eating that feels better to you.

[**BRITT:** When Sumner first told me to give myself permission to eat my favorite foods again and to eat them without guilt, I was terrified. I thought guilt was the only thing that separated me from losing control. In fact, trying to eat without guilt made me feel like Sumner was sabotaging me. Of course, the opposite was true. By ditching the guilt, I ended up eating less and overall feeling more in control.]

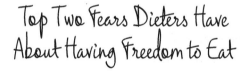

Top Two Fears Dieters Have About Having Freedom to Eat

#1 "I'll always choose to eat junk food."

#2 "I'll gain weight if I let myself eat what I want."

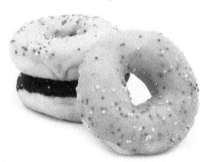

ABSTINENCE IS YOUR DOWNFALL

Believe it or not, totally cutting out certain foods is not necessary for weight loss. Plenty of diet-book authors and weight-loss plans are against you eating whatever you want, because it's more convincing and absolute to promise results if you tell someone they have to banish something forever. What you need to know to be smarter than all of the diet plans out there is that abstaining from something you need to feel satisfied will eventually backfire on you and create an urge to eat impulsively or binge.

Freedom to eat what you want is initially terrifying because you're worried that you'll only want to eat junk food. Yet what I see over and over again is that when a person gives herself the freedom to eat what she wants, she naturally craves a variety of foods—yes, even healthy foods. And, the best part is this: when you have permission to eat the foods you crave, they end up no longer having the same emotional pull on you as they did when they were forbidden.

Of course, having permission to eat anything you want doesn't mean you'll never crave junk food again. There will be times you will crave white truffle mac and cheese or freshly baked chocolate-chip cookies, and there will be other times you'll crave a big, juicy mango or veggie-filled salad. Think of your body as its own universe; it's always shifting to achieve a cosmic balance.

WATCH OUT FOR PSEUDO-PERMISSION

OK, so you've got the gist: You're going to let yourself eat all the foods you like. Forbidden foods? No such thing. However, if you tell yourself it's fine to have that double-dark chocolate cake after dinner—but then start calculating how many extra miles you have to run the next day—you've given yourself pseudo-permission (aka guilt in disguise). You need true, full, unconditional freedom to eat what sounds satisfying to you if this non-diet way of eating is going to work.

[BRITT: I'm going to throw myself under the bus for a second here because I really want you to understand how important it is to avoid pseudo-permission.

I was a total pseudo-permission giver when I first started working with Sumner. I understood the logic behind the no-diet plan, but I thought it would only work for Sumner's other clients. All I wanted was to be skinny, and a part of me couldn't grasp that I would actually look my best if I allowed myself to eat what I wanted. So I charged into Sumner's office one afternoon visibly upset. I told her I didn't buy into this philosophy and I wanted to take a break. Sumner was patient and kind and told me that she was there for me whenever I was ready to come back. She knew I'd be back.

Two months and another failed diet later, I called Sumner and told her I was ready to take this seriously and really try this "non-dieting thing." Once I finally let myself have full permission and let go of guilt about my food choices, change started to happen so fast it was exhilarating. And the best part was, I was having so much fun. Eating food became exciting, dining out was fun again, and guilt was nowhere to be found. Oh, and over a few weeks my pants started to fit a bit better too.]

INTUITIVE EATING WORKS

Studies clearly demonstrate that women with high Intuitive Eating Scale (IES) scores have significantly lower body mass index (BMI). This means people who trust their bodies and find ways to cope with their feelings without using food are less likely to engage in eating behaviors that lead to excess weight gain. There is no scientific evidence that shows restrictive diets lead to lasting weight loss or improved health parameters. In fact, research shows that following those kinds of diets is actually a predictor of weight gain.

FORGET ABOUT YOUR WEIGHT-LOSS GOAL—FOR NOW

If you are going to make the transition from being besties with Guilt and Shame to being a Savvy Eater, the first thing you need to do is forget about your weight-loss goal—at least at first. Yep, you heard that right: Your weight loss goal can't be front and center on your priority list. If it is, it can keep you from making progress.

Worrying about weight gain is a natural response. It takes time to ditch years of dieting thoughts and to transition to a healthier, long-term approach to eating and nourishing yourself. The only way you can learn to give yourself permission to eat is if you don't have a scale holding you to a number. In this process, weighing yourself every day is like trying to run with your shoelaces tied together. You just won't get anywhere.

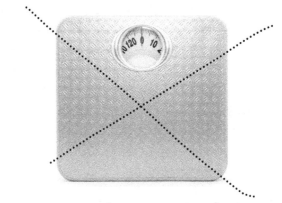

Take a minute right now and hide your scale. Out of sight, out of mind.

AIM FOR PROGRESS, NOT PERFECTION

Initially, you may feel compelled to eat more than you need, or eat more often than you truly want, because you're not totally sure this "freedom to eat" thing is going to last.

It's like you have to prove to yourself that you really can have what you want. It is totally normal to experience a desire to eat what you've been missing at almost every opportunity you have. Just keep in mind that you do not have to be perfect for this to work. Each time you have an experience that feels better for you is a win.

#ProgressNotPerfection

[BRITT: When I was dieting, I would order only skinny vanilla lattes at Starbucks and I would never let myself even think of ordering a treat. Treats and pastries were forbidden, since I was constantly in a state of trying to lose weight.

When I finally allowed myself permission to eat all foods, I went straight for the bright-pink birthday cake pops. Every time I went to Starbucks I would order that cake pop.

Eventually, I began to realize that I didn't always want a cake pop when I ordered my coffee. Then another lightbulb went off: just because I had permission to order something sweet, that didn't mean I needed to order it. Here was an even bigger shocker: the cake pop didn't even taste as good or feel as good in my body when I wasn't craving one. This made me realize that the way I thought about food was the root of my issues with food.]

THE SATISFYING TRUTH

Savvy Eaters eat the right amount of food for their bodies, have no guilt or judgment about what they eat, and they aim to feel completely satiated after a meal or snack. Eating to feel satisfied is essential because your body will start to trust that you're no longer going to be deprived, and that you don't have to eat anything impulsively anymore. This is when food starts to become emotionally neutral.

Two Types of Satisfaction

Leaving a meal feeling "satisfied" is a result of these two types of satisfaction.

PHYSICAL SATISFACTION

This means having enough calories and nourishment to feel comfortably full. Physical satisfaction is letting yourself have enough of what you want, not limiting it to the amount you think you "should" have, and involves feeling good physically after you eat the food.

EMOTIONAL SATISFACTION

This means getting pleasure from eating food. Finding emotional satisfaction from your food relates to having enjoyed the flavors, textures, tastes, appearance, and temperature of what you ate. Essentially, you feel that you ate what you really wanted.

A SAVVY EATER IS A SATISFIED EATER

Ask yourself these questions before meals to help yourself become a more satisfied eater.

Q: HOW DO I WANT TO FEEL AFTER I FINISH EATING?

A: Answering this question is a major part of feeling satisfied, comfortable, and content with your food choices. Pay attention to how different foods make you feel and what amount of food feels best. Cut back on the foods that don't make you feel great and fully enjoy the foods that make you feel good and give you energy.

[BRITT: Pizza is one of my favorite foods. When I learned to give myself permission to eat it again I remember ordering pizza from the fast-food place near my apartment. I ate it without guilt, but afterward I felt a little sick—and not from overeating. After more pizza-eating experimenting (the best kind of science), I realized that pizza, when made from high-quality ingredients, made me feel great. Whereas greasy, fast-

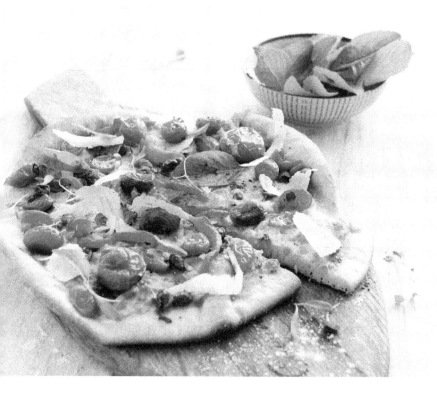

food pizza gave me a stomachache. The most amazing lesson for me here was the realization that my body intuitively knows what's better for me. I just have to be savvy enough to listen to the signals.]

Q: HOW MUCH OF THIS FOOD DO I NEED TO FEEL SATISFIED?

A: Eating to feel satisfied may not be what you're used to doing. If you love spaghetti and every time you eat it you automatically help yourself to an extra portion and then feel sluggish after your meal, you're probably eating too much of it. In this case, there's an issue of quantity. It's up to you to figure out how you can adjust the portion of that meal so that you enjoy it fully and feel good afterward.

FOOD FOR THOUGHT:

It is possible to be physically full but not satisfied.

Q: WHAT AM I HUNGRY FOR?

A: Have you ever finished a meal feeling a comfortable level of fullness but still found yourself on the prowl for more? In the past, if I told myself I was just going to fill up on protein and salad for dinner, I would never really feel satisfied. Then, the rest of my evening was spent on the hunt for something yummier, starchier, or sweeter. If you find yourself fantasizing about your next meal or snack almost immediately after finishing breakfast, lunch, or dinner, you may not be feeling adequately satisfied. Remember, your body knows what it needs, and one way or another it's going to ask for it.

Keep in Mind

FULLNESS—is how your stomach feels with the amount of food you ate or drank.

SATISFACTION—is getting enough of what you really want.

Next Up

➔ Are you an emotional eater? (Hint: you'll be surprised.)

➔ How to say no to food pushers

➔ A three-step process to prevent emotional eating

The Sneaky Reason you're Eating More than you Need

[BRITT: Giving myself permission to eat what I wanted took me a long time to fully embrace. Even after I started eating all the foods I wanted, I occasionally found myself eating too much of something extra-tasty.

For instance, one night my husband and I ordered sushi for dinner and I got a vegetable tempura roll. After eating some appetizers, I turned to the tempura roll. The first two or three pieces tasted amazing—the warm tempura was sweet and savory and I felt completely consumed by it. Before I knew it, I was stuffing the last piece in my mouth. Ten minutes later, I plopped myself on the couch in a food coma. The experience made me feel frustrated because I thought I was doing the right thing—giving myself permission to eat what I wanted instead of what I thought I should eat—but it tasted so good I couldn't stop myself.

"You see," I said to Sumner, half-ashamed at my lack of willpower, "I can't do this non-diet stuff, because I always end up uncomfortably full after eating yummy foods. Therefore I need a forbidden-foods list." What she told me next I would have never seen coming.

Sumner replied, "Well, let's take a step back. If you knew you were already full after the third piece, why do you think you kept eating? There is most certainly a reason behind this behavior. Yes, it tastes good, but if you can have that sushi tomorrow, the next day, and every other day of your life, why eat in a way that makes you feel uncomfortable? Perhaps you're trying to escape something? What were you feeling in that moment? What thoughts were going through your head before you started the meal?"

At first I was confused. "I love my life!" I told her. "I have nothing to escape from." But as we dug into the circumstances of the sushi moment, everything started to become clear. My workday had been stressful, I hadn't finished everything on my to-do list, and I also felt anxiety over the week's upcoming tasks. When we discussed what my ideal day would look like, we concluded that I had unrealistic expectations of what I could accomplish in a day. No wonder I always felt stressed, sad, and frustrated at night, even though my life overall felt great. It all came down to being too hard on myself.

Not surprisingly, the days I was stressed to the max were the days I would clean my plate at dinner, because I was using food as a way to escape these feelings. I would "check out" from my negative feelings during the eating process. So, although I could tell that I was getting full after the first few pieces, I didn't want the fun experience to end because that would mean I would have to go back to hanging out with my not-so-fun feelings. The reality, of course, is that eating can't last forever, and I would eventually be stuck with my undesirable emotions in addition to being uncomfortably full.

Recognizing how emotional eating is causing you to overeat is the key to doing something about it. Sumner helped me see that understanding and recognizing the emotions that drive our eating is equally as important as getting rid of that list of forbidden foods.]

WHAT IS EMOTIONAL EATING?

It's time to take an honest look at why you're eating. Brittany's story is proof of how important it is to get in touch with the reasons why you're reaching for food. No matter how much freedom you give yourself when it comes to eating—or how quickly you de-friend Guilt and Shame—you may still be eating more food than you need if you're eating for reasons other than hunger.

Emotional eating is the biggest reason why we eat when we're not hungry, and the unintended consequences are weight gain and the frustration that comes along with it. Emotional eating can be obvious (think sad breakup followed by girl in her PJs plowing through a pint of mint chocolate chip) or it can be very subtle (you finish a sushi roll even if you're stuffed to the max). The reality is, most of us are completely clueless about the fact that we're eating for reasons other than hunger, and so we don't even realize we're eating food that we don't need.

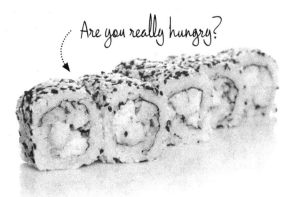

Are you really hungry?

The non-dieting approach works because we are dealing with the full picture of your eating. Once you develop the skills of being a Savvy Eater, it will become a way of life.

Emotional eating is so much more than just eating when we're sad. It can result from a wide variety of emotions (happiness, sadness, excitement, worry, stress) and automatic eating is often just the learned coping mechanism—it's how we check out and relax from a hard day's work or a tornado of uncomfortable feelings. Reading gossip magazines, binging on bad reality TV shows, having a good cry, watching Sex and the City marathons with your bestie, and even exercising are all coping mechanisms—and they only turn into trouble when they lead to undesirable behaviors or consequences.

There are lots of different emotions that might prompt you to eat. Think about the following scenarios and ask yourself if they've ever inspired you to overdo it.

Have you ever eaten to . . .

○ **AVOID** or procrastinate doing something you really don't want to do? Maybe you're avoiding opening a stack of overdue bills, washing the pile of dishes in the sink, doing four weeks' worth of laundry, finishing a super-boring work assignment, or even avoiding exercise?

○ **REWARD** yourself after a hard day, a good workout, or for an accomplishment?

○ **CELEBRATE** a holiday, birthday, new job, graduation, or Friday night with family and friends?

○ **PUNISH** yourself, either for making a mistake, upsetting someone, or even for eating something bad and feeling fat?

○ **ESCAPE** a feeling, such as stress, anxiety, anger, uncertainty, disappointment, or self-consciousness?

○ **RELAX** and unwind after a long day? Hello, wine, baguette, and cheese.

○ **COMFORT** yourself from sadness, depression, loneliness, hopelessness, or fear?

○ **ENTERTAIN** yourself, perhaps when bored by a task or not fulfilled in your life? Feeling empty? Nothing a little cookie dough can't fix, right?

○ **CONTINUE** feeling the pleasure of yummy food, even after you've had enough?

○ **JOIN** "The Clean Plate Club" and, like your parents taught you, never leave the table until you've finished your dinner?

○ **PLEASE** others at a dinner party, when the host gives you a slice of cake or an extra helping of food that you didn't want but ate anyway to make that person happy?

○ **AVOID** food waste by finishing the rest of yesterday's lasagna because you didn't want it to go in the garbage?

[BRITT: So, I think I've answered yes to all of these at some point—how about you? And I bet you didn't consider yourself an emotional eater before seeing this list . . . am I right?]

As you can see, there are many emotional reasons behind why we eat. When you get caught with an unpleasant feeling and reach for food out of habit, simply be aware of what you're doing.

One of my clients, Amy, wanted to talk to me about why she would eat more than she wanted to at parties. When we dug deeper, we found that she was automatically eating at social events because she felt self-conscious, and eating was a way of keeping herself occupied. Since Amy didn't consider herself a socially nervous person, it was hard for her to recognize that being around people she didn't know well triggered her to hover over the cheese platter. Instead, she'd always attributed her party eating to a lack of willpower.

Changing this behavior had to begin with an awareness of what was really going on. Challenging her old beliefs— that she wasn't worth talking to, didn't look pretty enough to approach new people, or didn't have anything interesting to say in a party situation—was an important first step.

I asked Amy if she could set herself up for success at an upcoming friend's barbecue. We set a plan that she would freely allow herself to eat any of the foods available if she felt hungry for them, but that she would not eat automatically as a way of keeping herself busy. Having that higher level of awareness—and a plan in place to be mindful of her body's hunger and fullness— worked so well, in fact, she reported back that she was "shocked." Awareness, and digging deeper to get to the root of the real problem, allowed Amy to discover that she actually didn't want to eat more food than felt comfortable to her. She realized that when she left the safety of the food table, she had the opportunity to sit and talk with interesting new people.

Amy knows now that she doesn't have to rely on food to protect her or keep her busy in social settings, and even though it was uncomfortable for her in the beginning, she made a big effort to be present at parties and to create real connections with people instead of focusing on the food at an event. The best part? In addition to coming home satisfied, Amy had the new confidence that she was perfectly fine showing up and being herself.

The bottom line is that we experience a lot of emotions on a daily basis, and we can't always control our emotions. We can control our reaction to them. By checking in regularly, you can train your brain to get in tune with what you're going through so you can choose to react in a way that feels best for you, rather than just reacting by eating on autopilot.

WHY IT MAY GET WORSE BEFORE IT GETS BETTER

The trade-off for feeling your not-so-fun feelings (which, by the way, we all have—it's just that we don't Instagram them) is that you learn how to process and tolerate them. You will strengthen your ability to give yourself what you really need instead of turning to food. It is incredibly liberating and empowering, but early on it may feel really crappy to notice all the negative emotions and actually face them.

I often give my clients a "homework" assignment: For one

week, write down the times when you allow yourself to feel and tolerate an uncomfortable emotion instead of turning to food. This is the point in the behavior change when you know what you're doing and you know it doesn't work well for you, but you actually have to push yourself to try a different coping mechanism. You will be amazed at how often you were running from something that you could've handled by facing it all along.

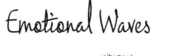

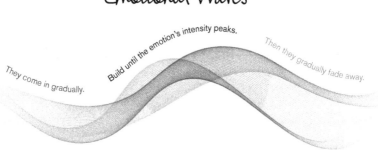

Visualize yourself riding the wave of the emotion.
Think to yourself: I'm strong enough to tolerate this emotion of boredom, sadness, loneliness, etc., and I know it will eventually pass.

WHY IGNORING YOUR FEELINGS WON'T WORK LONG-TERM

Instead of dealing with our feelings in a constructive way, many of us tend to bury our emotions deep within us. But we all know that suppressed emotions build up over time and eventually burst free one way or another. Have you ever had tensions with a friend and instead of calling her and working it out, you both ignored it, only to have it resurface later and become a way bigger issue?

Many of the people who walk through my door experience

buried emotions that come out through their eating. However, not everyone's stifled emotions manifest this way. Some deal with anger-management issues, drug and alcohol abuse, overworking, perfectionism, shopping, or even self-harm. Eating is a very common way for people to cope with feelings that aren't being addressed because it's cheap, legal, socially acceptable, quick, and readily available.

That said, sometimes you may eat something just for the emotion of pleasure. You may just want a fresh baked cookie right out of the oven for no other reason than it is delicious. There is nothing wrong with that and, in fact, it's a normal desire. It is not necessary, nor realistic, to expect that every time you eat will only be strictly because you're hungry.

HOW TO DEAL WITH A FOOD PUSHER

Maybe your parents were the first food pushers, nudging you to eat all of your veggies. Then, maybe your best friend's mom liked to plop another piece of her famous apple pie in front of you once you were finished with your first slice. Now as an adult, it may even be a friend who wants all of her spinach dip gone before all of the guests leave her party so that she herself isn't tempted to eat it. Keep in mind, only you can know when you want or need to put something in your body, and it's a personal decision—one that shouldn't be influenced by anyone else. If you feel it's polite to eat something in order to show your gratitude or appreciation, remember that you can show that with words—not with your fork. Here are a few examples of what to say . . .

▶ "No, thank you. I wish I had more room, but I'm already full!"

▶ "That looks amazing! Thank you for making this. May I take one home for later?"

▶ "I appreciate you treating me to this lovely meal—it's been absolutely amazing. I wish I had more room for all of it."

▶ "I really won't feel well if I eat more, but thank you. It's delicious."

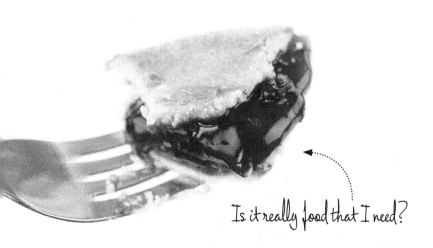

Is it really food that I need?

THREE STEPS TO DEALING WITH YOUR FEELINGS (INSTEAD OF EATING TO COPE OR DISTRACT YOURSELF)

STEP 1: BE AWARE OF EMOTIONAL EATING

ASK YOURSELF: "AM I PHYSICALLY HUNGRY?"

If the answer is yes, then ask, "What do I want? How much do I need? What will feel satisfying?" Make the food you need, put it on a plate, and sit down so you can really taste and enjoy your meal.

If the answer is no, then ask, "What am I feeling?" Express the feeling or emotion with as much detail as you possibly can.

THEN ASK YOURSELF: "WHAT IS IT THAT I REALLY NEED, AND CAN I GIVE MYSELF WHAT I REALLY NEED?"

If yes, do it! Allow yourself to do what you really want in that moment. (Are you working and need a break? You don't have to eat to take a break.).

If no, ask yourself: "How can I help myself deal with this feeling if I can't have what I really need?"

STEP 2: COMMIT TO HELPING YOURSELF GET THROUGH THE FEELING

PROCESS WHAT YOU'RE FEELING:

▸ Call a friend.

▸ Journal for a few minutes.

▸ Talk to yourself about what's going on.

▸ Write a hypothetical e-mail to someone even if you don't press Send.

▸ Make a therapy appointment.

[BRITT: Therapy is not for the weak. I've been, and I love it. Sometimes it's really nice to have a third party to talk to about life, to get validation about how you feel, and to get those buried emotions out of you. Even if you only go for a session or two, you will (usually) feel a bit better afterward.]

DISTRACT OR SOOTHE:

▸ Read a book.

▸ Go for a walk or exercise.

▸ Take a yoga class.

▸ Start a DIY project.

▸ Organize your photos or create a photo book.

▸ Drive to a pretty place and just sit with your thoughts.

SIT BACK AND RELAX:

▸ Listen to music or make a new playlist.

▸ Watch TV, a movie, or a TED talk.

▸ Meditate or lie down and rest.

▸ Take a bath or hot shower.

▸ Book a massage.

TAKE ACTION TOWARD RESOLVING WHAT'S BOTHERING YOU:

If you're worried about a project or a daunting task, for example, take one step toward starting it. Simply make a plan or an outline, or do fifteen minutes of work and then give yourself permission to reevaluate the situation.

If you're beating yourself up for a mistake, forgive yourself, then see if there's anything you can do to apologize, correct, or fix what happened. You can't change the past; all you can do is learn from it. So, look for the lesson, keep a positive attitude, and move forward.

savvy tip

Make sure your to-do list has "actionable" items instead of abstract actions. For example, if "write a book" is on your to-do list, that task can be daunting. Instead, make smaller, more actionable items, such as write a chapter, or simply write for two hours. You may feel unsure about how to write a book, but you definitely know how to write for two hours.

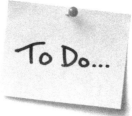

STEP 3: DON'T BEAT YOURSELF UP, NO MATTER WHAT HAPPENED (OR WHAT YOU ATE)

Change your thoughts and you will change your life. Our thoughts become our words, and our words become our actions. This is why if you have a binge or an emotional-eating experience and beat yourself up about it, those negative thoughts will result in more negative behavior. Reflect on what happened in an emotionally neutral way and consider what you'd like to do differently next time. Savvy Girls don't wallow in guilt and shame; instead, they follow this thought pattern:

A recent experience that I would do differently is _____ _____.

I was feeling _____ when I was going through it.

I didn't have _____ that would've helped me.

Instead of turning to food and comfort eating, I would have rather _____.

Change happens when you become aware of the self-talk going on in your head. If you notice you're beginning to eat in a way that you feel is not for hunger, here are some examples of questions and statements you can think about to help neutralize the negative thoughts that make you eat more:

▸ I'm going to take two minutes and pause to feel my hunger level. I have permission to keep eating if that's what I choose.

▸ I have permission to eat this food, so why am I eating it so fast, or too much of it, or so impulsively?

▸ Is there an emotion or feeling I'm trying to escape right now?

▸ How am I going to feel in thirty minutes if I eat this food for emotional reasons?

▸ What is the worst part about the feeling I'm running from?

▸ I deserve to feel good in my body, so why would I eat in a way that doesn't end up feeling good for me?

▸ What have I learned from the past about how it works for me to eat in this way?

▸ I do not expect myself to be perfect—it's not necessary or realistic.

▸ I don't need to beat myself up; this is not about food.

▸ Is it possible for me to give myself what I really need, since I know I'm not hungry?

Remember: Your goal is to focus on progress, not perfection—especially when it comes to changing your eating habits. It's normal and expected that you won't be able to change every automatic or emotional eating impulse right away. It's critical for you to forgive yourself for any uncomfortable eating experiences and try to learn from them. I always tell my clients, "Every binge has a message." Over time, the positive outcomes will build a new memory bank of Savvy Eating experiences, which will motivate you to continue your new, non-dieting way of thinking about food.

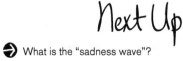

Next Up

→ What is the "sadness wave"?

→ How to determine when to stop eating without feeling deprived

→ Tips for keeping your "hangry" moments in check

The Secret to Never Counting Calories Again

[BRITT: I'm going to go ahead and do what every other self-help book doesn't: I'm going to give you the secret of this chapter right here, at the very start:

"The secret to never counting calories again is mastering when to eat and when you've had enough by becoming aware of where your hunger and fullness falls on the Hunger and Fullness Spectrum," says Sumner. "To do that, you must get back in touch with learning how to hear your personal hunger and fullness cues."

There you have it. Eat when you're hungry, stop when you're full. I don't know about you, but I've found doing this to be a lot harder than it sounds.

Think about how many times you've sat on the couch after Thanksgiving, jeans unbuttoned, solemnly swearing off turkey feasts for good . . . or until next year, that is. If we could really trust our bodies to tell us when we've had enough, why would we ever let ourselves get so sickly full on that last Thursday in November?

Or how about the ravenous hunger that creeps up on us out of nowhere? The "I need to eat right NOW, or I will hurt someone"—type of hunger. The word "hangry" was created for a reason.

And what about the times our hunger and fullness is less obvious? Say, when you're looking down at your turkey sandwich and you think: To eat the second half, or not to eat the second half? That is the question. As if this decision were a question philosophers have pondered for millennia.

Or what about when you finish a delicious dinner at your favorite restaurant, you're full, and you know you don't want another bite. But it's your friend's birthday dinner and someone passes you a slice of cake and before you know it, you inhale that sugary slice of red-velvet heaven. And as your last bite pulls you back to Earth, you wonder how you could have possibly been hungry for dessert when mere minutes before you knew you couldn't have another bite of dinner?

When our bodies send us confusing signals like this, how the heck are we supposed to trust our bodies to count calories for us? Enter Sumner, who has developed an easy way to better grasp our hunger and fullness cues so we can go back to trusting our bodies to do the calorie-counting work for us.]

You'll probably be surprised by how simple, yet eye-opening, the Hunger and Fullness Spectrum really is—it's the same reaction the majority of my clients have. For many dieters, counting calories and watching carbs seems to make way more sense (initially) than listening to their bodies.

A client once asked me, "So, are you telling me that calories don't matter at all?" She was confused. I told her that calories do matter, but that we don't need to count them. Your body and brain are designed to essentially count calories for you. When we need more calories, we need to eat more to feel satisfied; when we need fewer cals, our hunger will calm down.

Don't worry—I'm going to go over these signals in detail (and why they can get confusing at times) so you can get out of your own way and trust that your body's got it covered.

HOW TO HEAR YOUR HUNGER AND FULLNESS

I know what you're thinking: If it's so simple to listen to our body, why doesn't everyone do it?

The reason? As a culture, we are more focused on accomplishing tasks and getting from one place to the next than we are on slowing down and enjoying a good meal. The faster and more distracted you are while eating, the less likely you are to hear your hunger and fullness signals. Also, people are used to not trusting their bodies because the dieting mentality has convinced them that they can't be trusted and that they'll never be thin enough—so the need to count calories and follow food rules has become the norm.

The good news: Those confusing signals can actually be cleared up easily by using the Hunger and Fullness Spectrum.

Take a minute to check in with what level of physical hunger or fullness you are experiencing right now. Start by asking yourself, Do I feel any hunger or fullness? Use this visual to help you identify what your body is telling you.

After checking in with your body, is it easy or difficult for you to gauge your current fullness or hunger? Where did you put yourself on the spectrum?

savvy tip [Snack when you have a low level of hunger. Snacks are designed to help fuel you and keep you comfortable and functioning until your next meal.]

Don't worry if you're a little unsure at the moment. Brittany was the same way when she first started learning to listen to her hunger and fullness levels. After years of eating when it was her scheduled time to eat, she had lost touch with what the low-to-medium hunger and fullness levels felt like. The goal here is not

Hunger and Fullness Spectrum

HUNGER

HIGH	MEDIUM	LOW
ravenous, low-blood sugar, high cravings	meal hungry	slightly hungry

to focus on how hungry or full you think you should be based on when you last ate (remember—ditch the shoulds!), but to listen to what your body is telling you in the present moment and trust it.

Also, keep in mind that there is no right or wrong level of hunger or fullness. The purpose of this spectrum is to help you realize that hunger and fullness is not black or white—it's a gradient—so becoming aware of where you are on this gradient will help you know whether you actually want the second half of your sandwich or whether you may want to consider slowing down or pausing during your meal so you don't accidentally get to a point where you feel uncomfortably full.

[BRITT: After a little practice, I stopped watching my weight and started letting my body worry about weight management. Listening to my body's signals is so much easier than trying to pre-portion my meals into the amount of food I think I should eat.]

STOP COMPARING YOURSELF TO OTHERS

Have you ever gone to lunch with a friend and felt uneasy or guilty for eating your whole meal while your friend barely touched her salad? From this day on, don't worry about it! Maybe your friend had a huge breakfast. Or maybe she has early dinner plans. Or maybe she just had a Frappuccino, which spoiled her appetite. No

FULLNESS

LOW	MEDIUM	HIGH
hunger is gone but not much fullness	comfortably full	uncomfortably full, stuffed

ss

matter what the reason, you've got to keep in mind that your only job is to know what you need. If you start to adjust your eating to match someone else's or to please others, you're very likely to under- or overeat. It's unlikely that two people having lunch together are going to have exactly the same level of hunger and eat the same amount of food. Bottom line: Don't compare yourself to your dining companion. Just focus on your lovely self.

Not sure what to look for?

Common Signals of...

Medium Hunger

- ○ Food sounds appetizing.
- ○ You want to sit down to a meal.
- ○ You crave something specific.
- ○ You feel emptiness in your stomach.
- ○ You salivate when you think about eating.
- ○ You're watching the clock for when it's lunchtime.

High Hunger

- ○ You have trouble concentrating.
- ○ You want to eat a lot.
- ○ You have a desire to eat fast.
- ○ You have a very empty stomach feeling, as well as hunger pains.
- ○ You get irritated if you have to wait to eat.
- ○ Your stomach is growling.
- ○ Your body temperature may change.
- ○ You have low energy, you feel tired, and/or you get a headache.
- ○ You're moody and short on patience.

Medium Fullness

- ○ You can feel food in your stomach.
- ○ You would not feel deprived if you stopped eating.
- ○ Your feeling of hunger is gone.
- ○ You feel indifferent toward food.
- ○ You notice food doesn't taste as good as when you started.

High Fullness

- ○ You have a "food baby" (your stomach is distended).
- ○ You're in a food coma (you find it hard to be productive or active).
- ○ There's pressure in your stomach
- ○ You feel sick, lethargic, and/or sleepy.
- ○ Your energy plummets.
- ○ It doesn't feel physically good to keep eating, despite taste.

YOU'RE THE BOSS!

Dieters are constantly either being "good" and sticking to the rules or they're being "bad" and rebelling by eating all kinds of foods they've deemed off-limits. Wouldn't you love to be the boss of what, when, and how much you eat and not have to be "good" or "bad" ever again? One of the best parts of switching to a non-dieting approach to eating is that you get to be in charge again. You get to decide when it feels best for you to start and stop eating.

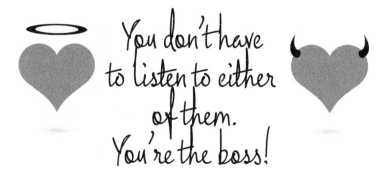

You don't have to listen to either of them. You're the boss!

When you're the boss, there is no one to rebel against. If it doesn't feel good for you to finish a meal and feel overly full, you can set your intention to stop when you've reached a medium level of fullness. No more feeling that you're either "good" or "bad" for stopping, even if everyone else is still eating. (Remember, they may not be listening to their fullness signals.)

And if you know that waiting until you're ravenous to eat usually leads to overeating, try eating earlier, when you have low or medium hunger, or stash a few snacks in your desk drawer or car glove box so you're prepared. When you start eating at times that feel right—and stop when you feel a comfortable level of fullness—a level of trust between your mind, body, and food begins to develop. And this, I can promise you, means never needing to count calories again.

TRUST YO'SELF

There is so much fear involved in dieting: fear of food, fear of never getting enough of the foods you love, fear of gaining weight, fear of failing again. I know at this point it's hard to imagine being that girl who can eat what she wants when she's hungry and stop when she's had enough. But that is what happens over and over again when dieters give themselves permission to eat.

When you eat what you really want and eat according to hunger and fullness, you'll naturally stop feeling afraid that you'll eat too much when something delicious crosses your path. Remember, one of the main reasons you feel out of control or like you can't stop at the right point of fullness is because in your subconscious dieting mind, you think you can't have that food again. When your brain realizes that you're not going to swear off pizza again, you can begin to trust yourself. You'll begin to fully believe that you're done swearing off anything that tastes good and, as a result, you'll be less inclined to eat a few extra slices even though you're full.

savvy tip [Download Sumner's Mindful Meal Timer and Mindful Meal Trainer apps on your phone to help you practice slowing down and checking in while eating.]

THE SCIENCE BEHIND WHEN TO STOP EATING

So, how does your stomach tell your brain to stop eating? It's a pretty amazing and complex communication system, the details of which I won't bore you with here. However, these two components of the process are worth knowing:

1. Stretch receptors that feel food in your stomach signal your brain that you're full.

2. A signal is sent from digestive hormones in the gastrointestinal tract that you've had enough food, which can take 20 to 30 minutes.

This is why slowing down when you eat is crucial if you're trying to hear your fullness before it's too late. When you eat fast because you're ravenous, your body's "I'm full now" message is still taking its sweet ol' time to get to your brain. So if you don't want to hit "Thanksgiving stuffed" and later regret it, slooooooow down!

Ditto when it comes to eating when you're distracted. Watching TV or shoveling in your Whole Foods salad while you check e-mail makes it nearly impossible to be present as you're eating. How will you know when you've had enough if you weren't paying attention? Put your health first and sit down to eat your meals without distractions so you can be mindful and pay attention to your hunger and fullness cues.

ALWAYS HUNGRY? HOW NUTRITION AFFECTS WHAT YOU HEAR

Did you know that the quality of the food you eat plays a big role in the loudness of your hunger and fullness signals? Without getting caught up in food rules, all you need to know is that when your body is receiving the calories, vitamins, minerals, fibers, and antioxidants it needs, it's better nourished. And when your body is better nourished, it sends you accurate hunger and fullness signals.

I'm not saying that everything you eat has to be nutritious; I am saying that eating mostly foods that lack quality nutrition does have a higher likelihood of causing you to feel constantly hungry. Why? When you eat low-nutrient junk foods, and low-cal diet foods, the body knows that it's not getting nourished. The result?

It'll keep asking you for more food, despite the amount of calories you may be consuming. Your body does not care if your little black dress won't zip; it wants its nutrition!

Don't get me wrong, here—if you want something sweet after dinner, go ahead and have it. That's different from eating only sweets all day and expecting to get clear hunger and fullness signals. Also, if you feel like you feed yourself nourishing foods and you still feel hungry all the time, it's possible you're either eating for emotional reasons or you are not eating the right foods in the right quantities to feel satisfied.

POORLY NOURISHED BODY = MIXED, INACCURATE HUNGER/ FULLNESS SIGNALS

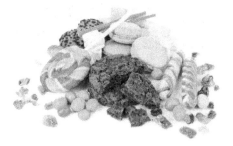

WELL-NOURISHED BODY = CLEAR AND ACCURATE SIGNALS

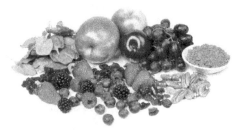

WHEN IS ENOUGH ENOUGH?

As you learn how to gauge your hunger and fullness, you'll also begin to discover your last-bite threshold (LBT), a concept of Intuitive Eating. The LBT is the point when you consciously decide you're nearing your desired fullness level and your next bite will be your last. Of course, you can always have more if you decide you need it, but identifying your LBT is a great way to eat mindfully.

[BRITT: It took me a while to discover my LBT because my comfortable fullness level occurs a few minutes after passing my last bite threshold. As a result, I learned to stop eating a touch earlier than I really wanted to, knowing that my fullness would set in shortly. At first it was torturous to not take those extra few bites, but in the long run, I've felt happier eating just a little bit less. My last-bite threshold isn't very loud—it's more of a soft knock—so learning to get comfortable with it, and to trust it, was empowering.]

Getting used to finding your LBT can feel like aiming at a moving dart board at times, so don't expect it to be a cinch. The more mindfully you eat and the more you practice tuning in to your hunger, the sooner you will consistently hit the bull's-eye.

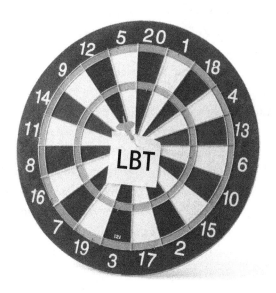

Also, don't forget to focus on making progress toward hitting your LBT instead of striving for perfection. There will be times when you forget to pay attention, or something else in life will attract more of your focus and you'll find yourself reverting to an old behavior, such as eating too fast or eating everything on your plate just because it's there. If this happens, be patient with yourself and don't judge yourself (hitting a bull's-eye is harder than it looks!). To keep focused on progress and not perfection, observe why you might have overeaten, learn from it, and move on.

THERE'S A REASON WE LOVE TOO MUCH OF A GOOD THING

We've all reached the bottom of that Girl Scout cookie box at some point or another. When we eat something delicious, we don't want it to end. A big part of why you may feel it's hard to stop eating something that tastes good when you know you've had enough is that it's sad—yes, sad—to end the eating experience. Think of this as the same type of sadness as when your vacation is over. It's sad when something good ends.

One of the original Intuitive Eating Pros, Elyse Resch, taught me that feeling sad is an emotion we need to learn to tolerate if we want to master the art of stopping at the right place. If you keep eating beyond what you need just to avoid feeling that sadness, you'll end up feeling worse. You'll feel frustrated with yourself or simply that uncomfortable fullness that makes you want to put on your "not tonight" sweatpants and crash on the couch.

Picture your eating experience as climbing a mountain: Visualize reaching the top of the mountain, when you've enjoyed as much of the meal as possible. Every food experience peaks, and if you keep eating you won't get any more enjoyment. If you continue past the "peak" when you're eating, the food may still taste good but your eating experience will start to turn negative. That's because you're eating beyond what your body needs, and that never feels good in the end.

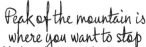
Peak of the mountain is where you want to stop
Maxium pleasure, enjoyment, and
satisfaction is found here. Continuing to
eat won't add to your enjoyment.

Getting closer
to satisfaction

Eating past the peak
may create a negative
eating experience

Enjoyable eating experience
Still have room for food.
You're not ready to stop yet.

savvy tip

Try "TAKING 10." If you feel sad that you're getting full but there is still more delicious food to eat, take a break for ten to twenty minutes. If you're still hungry for more after that time-out is up, go for it. Just knowing that you can have seconds in twenty minutes makes the sadness wave more bearable. Why the seemingly random ten-to-twenty-minute mark? That's typically when we can physically feel our fullness.

QUICK TIPS FOR WHEN YOU'RE "HANGRY"

Although it's ideal to eat when you're at a medium hunger level, try not to panic if you get to a ravenous level. Sometimes it creeps up on us, and sometimes we just get busy and don't get a moment to squeeze in a meal. Here are some of my best tips on how to stay savvy when hungry gets hangry:

1. Set an intention. How do you want to feel when you're done eating? Be mindful of your goal to reach a comfortable level of fullness and remind yourself that as soon as you get even a few bites of something into your body, you will calm down and feel better.

2. Go for carbs. If you can find food with carbohydrates (crackers, fruit, granola bar, bread, pretzels, etc.), it will help to raise your blood sugar (which plummeted when you were super-hungry) and help you regain your senses. Only carbs quickly raise your blood sugar; they're also your brain's preferred fuel source. If you reach for protein, it won't give your body the physiological rise in blood sugar that it needs to feel good again. (Ideally, have that carb with some protein and fat for good blood sugar control.)

3. Slow down. After a few bites, set down your fork, take a short break, and remind yourself that you can eat as much as you need to feel satisfied. Don't forget to listen for that LBT.

MASTERING THE HUNGER SPECTRUM BY PLANNING AHEAD

If you know you've got a flurry of meetings for the next five hours after a meal, you may want to eat to a higher level of fullness than if you were going to be able to have a snack in two to three hours when your hunger spectrum shifts to "light" hunger. It's perfectly useful—and necessary—to allow yourself to use your head when deciding how much to eat. Your ultimate job is to keep yourself comfortable, content, and nourished. Thinking ahead can help.

Quick and Easy Foods to Keep on Hand:

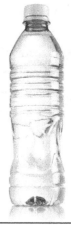

- Cheese and crackers
- Peanut-butter sandwich
- Apple and trail mix or nut butter
- Yogurt and dry cereal
- Snack bars with carbs, protein, and fat
- Turkey and cheese on English muffin
- Dry-roasted soybeans with fresh fruit
- Hard-boiled eggs and cut vegetables
- 1 oz. dark chocolate and almonds or pistachios
- A bottle of water to keep you hydrated

WHAT TO DO WHEN YOU DON'T FOLLOW THAT (AWESOME) ADVICE . . .

If you have an eating experience that doesn't feel good, here are some questions to ask yourself that'll help you stay out of the dieting cycle:

- ▸ What would I rather do differently next time?

- ▸ Did I feel deprived of something?

- ▸ When or why did I forget to listen to my hunger and fullness levels?

- ▸ Was I eating for emotional reasons rather than physical hunger?

You don't need to feel guilty about what happened, but it is a good idea to understand what led to you making the decision you did, and how you can learn from the scenario.

Most important, remind yourself that your body will take care of any prior overeating naturally, by adjusting your hunger level later (remember, your body and brain are designed to monitor these things). Whatever you do, don't deprive yourself or double up on exercise to try to "undo" an eating choice that you regret. One meal or one day of eating never changed anyone's body. So, if you ate something that you regret or forgot to honor your fullness signals, you haven't ruined anything. It's how you interpret the experience and learn from it that matters most. Your thought patterns are key to having a healthy relationship with food.

Next Up

⮑ Does exercise help you lose weight?

⮑ How many days a week do you need to exercise?

⮑ Do you have to sweat for your workout to count?

Exercise Does Not Make you Lose Weight (gasp!)

[BRITT: At one of my sessions with Sumner I asked, "Should I be worried if I hate exercise?" I had just come from an intense Pilates class, where I had struggled to make it through to the end. I almost didn't finish that class, not due to physical exhaustion, but rather because I was mentally pooped. I had reached a point where I just couldn't force myself to listen to another instructor count to a hundred as my abs burned, and that realization terrified me.

After telling Sumner about how sure I was that I never wanted to see a Pilates reformer again, she suggested that I take a break from exercise altogether. "Don't do any exercise you don't want to do," she told me.

"What? Are you serious? For how long?" I asked.

"However long you want, whether that is a week, six months, or indefinitely," she said. "Just make sure to observe how you feel, and see if you can find the amount of activity that feels best for you."

I felt like a kid whose teacher actually told her to skip school. I was thrilled. Adios, Pilates; hello, couch. For the first week or so I did absolutely nothing. It felt glorious for the first few days (a sign my body probably needed the rest), but by the end of the third week, the "blah-ness" was starting to set in. I actually wanted to move around, but I definitely did not want to go back to Pilates.

Wanting to feel better, I started going on long walks. The intensity was perfect and the movement felt great. After a few more weeks, I started playing tennis and I went on hikes—but I didn't touch a barbell or set foot into a fitness studio for several months.

The craziest thing is my weight did not change much from the period of time I was doing lots of intense exercise where I hated every moment of it, versus doing no exercise at all. This

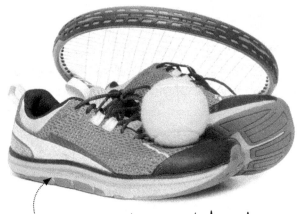

Getting active because it feels good is the best motivator

gave me mixed feelings. On one hand it felt great that I didn't need to wake up at six a.m. to have my ass kicked in order to maintain my weight. At the same time, I felt a bit of regret that I had spent so many years dragging myself to punishing workouts in hopes of losing weight when the reality was it wasn't making a difference. To think of all of the "working out" dread I could have avoided, the extra sleep I could have enjoyed, and the extra dollars I would have saved if I had known that exercise doesn't make you lose weight.

The thing about exercise is that being "active" does feel good, and it is part of a healthy lifestyle. The catch? This is true only if you find a form of exercise that feels good for you. And that is what this chapter is all about—learning to reframe your perspective on exercise and to find the type of activity and amount of activity that is right for you. Exercise needs to add to your life instead of detract from it, and in this chapter we are going to show you how to find the right balance.]

When I was a chronic dieter, I was also a compulsive exerciser. Some days I'd spend hours in the dingy basement of the local gym, telling myself I wasn't allowed to leave until I'd burned 2,000 calories or sometimes even more. I know . . . so absurd. My goal was to burn off all of the calories in the food I ate earlier (and ideally more) so I was sure I'd lose weight.

I didn't lose weight.

I was a nutrition student with a lot of shame about my eating, so I felt compelled to exercise. In my mind, it was the only thing keeping me from gaining weight. It's so sad to look back and realize I was wasting hours of my life in that overly fluorescent gym when I was just blocks away from the beautiful San Diego beaches.

When I was stuck in my old dieting pattern, I would find myself eating as much as I wanted with no regard to my body's hunger or fullness signals. The plan was to burn it all off at the gym later . . . or so I thought. What I didn't realize then is how this was the perfect way to stay stuck in an emotional eating and bingeing rut. As long as I could work off the calories I consumed, I didn't have to deal with the emotions and feelings that were making me eat more than I needed in the first place.

DEFINITION: ACTIVITY DISORDER

I was using exercise as a way to build self-esteem, to justify eating, and to control my body and my life. This is known as activity disorder, and is also called exercise addiction, compulsive exercise, or exercise bulimia. These are all very serious psychological conditions that require professional therapy to heal. Serious damage, such as loss of menstruation, fatigue, adrenal exhaustion, muscle wasting and injury, depression, stress fractures, and osteoporosis can all happen to an exercise addict. Yes, serious stuff.

The thing is, I have always loved being active, but back then I didn't have the first clue about what it meant to love myself. I was constantly using exercise as a way to control my weight, thinking, The more I work out, the more weight I'll lose; then I'll be able to accept myself. As you can imagine—and what you may be experiencing yourself—is that exercising in this way does not make you lose weight or help you find more self-acceptance.

When you use exercise purely for burning calories, it becomes a way of giving yourself pseudo-permission to eat. There are two outcomes to this approach:

1. You don't give yourself permission to eat if you haven't exercised.

2. You eat more when you exercise more, because you think you can and also because you're actually more hungry.

What I've seen countless times with clients is that exercising for weight loss alone will not help you become a more active or fit person. If you become dependent on trying to burn off everything you're eating to manage your weight, you've missed the point of being a Savvy Eater, and you're putting yourself back on the dieting hamster wheel.

YOUR ACTIVITY LEVEL WILL DICTATE YOUR HUNGER

What I've learned—and what many of my clients feel relieved to discover—is that your appetite eventually shifts to match your activity level. Every time I have a client who is patiently healing from an injury and isn't able to do her normal activities, she notices a decline in her appetite during the time of non-activity. And that shift in hunger is often so natural and so gradual, she may not even realize it's happened until I ask. I've also seen many times that when someone exercises a lot on a regular basis, she will have a greater appetite. Her body will know to turn up the signals that ask for more food.

WHY THE ALL-OR-NOTHING APPROACH TO EXERCISE SUCKS

One of the biggest mistakes I see most dieters make is increasing their exercise at the same time they start trying to be "really healthy" (aka, when they start imposing serious calorie restriction on themselves). This is the classic New Year's resolution pitfall.

Why do most New Year's resolutions flop by February?

According to a study published in the Journal of Clinical Psychology, resolutions are a way of procrastinating. This makes total sense when you think about it. Why does everyone wait until January 1 to start making changes if they're supposedly so ready for a change? The study also found that one of the main reasons for such high rates of failure with resolutions is that people set out with unrealistic goals and expectations. By the following December, many people are back to where they started—or oftentimes, even worse off.

The short-lived nature of most weight-loss resolutions is a direct result of what happens to our hunger levels when we reduce our caloric intake while simultaneously increasing our exercise levels. If increased exercise means your body needs more calories to sustain itself—but you're not allowing yourself to eat—then you've got a perfect recipe for fatigue, deprivation, cravings, and depression. And there's a good chance that this combo is going to lead to you falling off your new plan.

Exercising specifically to lose weight ignores the reasons why we might want to be active other than for the purpose of weight loss, such as feeling better, happier, stronger, and more energized. When it's all about weight loss, how could exercising not feel like a chore?

GETTING ACTIVE VS. OBLIGATORY EXERCISE

"How do you feel if you don't move?"

This is the question I asked Brittany when she asked about the minimum amount of exercise she needed to do. It's a question I often ask clients who are struggling with guilt if they don't work out or fear of gaining weight if they miss their workout.

I'll encourage them to try to be nonjudgmental, and instead curiously look at how they feel if they stop moving much for a few days or a week.

Like Brittany, most clients come back after a period of not doing obligatory exercise and tell me that they actually feel better, more energized, and have clearer hunger signals when they move regularly in a way that they enjoy. I then ask them, "Are these newfound benefits things that you value? Are they reasons why you might be motivated to move your body because you choose to, instead of moving your body just for the sake of weight control?"

Take a minute now and answer these questions for yourself. You might realize you like being active more than you thought you did, and that you do want to move because it makes you feel good—not because it burns calories.

[BRITT: When Sumner told me weight loss usually isn't enough of a motivator to hit the gym, I thought that made no sense. I would never attend Pilates if it weren't for my desire for a small waistline. Who in the world would subject herself to "Pilates 100s" (aka the most intense sit-ups ever created) otherwise?

But then I started to remember my sporadic Pilates schedule. I would hit it hard with four Pilates classes in one week, then the following week I would have to force myself to attend three while dreading every minute of it. By the third week I would hit Snooze on my alarm clock and skip a few classes, and by the fourth week I was "too busy" to make it to any classes.

Hmmm . . . Sumner might be on to something. Weight loss was enough of a motivator to get me to a few classes in the beginning, but it wasn't enough of a motivator to keep me there. When it came down to another hour of sleep or another dreaded Pilates class, extra time with my pillow won every time. I mean, it wasn't even a fair fight.]

So, what is enough of a motivator to get up and move? The answer: feeling strong in your body, the positive mind-set you get from all of those happy-making endorphins, and improving your energy. Someone who enjoys moving is motivated to make getting active a part of her everyday routine because it makes her feel better and adds value to her life.

HOW IS "GETTING ACTIVE" DIFFERENT FROM EXERCISE?

Getting active is something we are designed to do. The human body needs to move to stay healthy, which is why it feels good when we are active, especially when it's balanced with enough rest. "Exercise" can be a toxic word to many chronic dieters because it often comes back to that feeling that it's something you have to do, not something you choose to do (kind of like those "Pilates 100s" for Brittany).

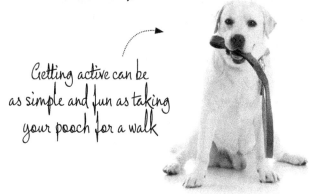

Getting active can be as simple and fun as taking your pooch for a walk

But here's a little secret that may change your life: You don't have to be at a gym running on a treadmill in order to move. Movement can be anything, from walking, swimming, or biking to playing with kids or animals, cleaning the house, or even running errands. Choose some form of movement that you enjoy; otherwise, you're not going to choose to do it regularly. If you finish a workout feeling energized, you're on the right track. When you're exhausted from vigorously overexercising and undereating, it's time for a new game plan.

THE TRUTH ABOUT CARBOHYDRATES AND EXERCISE

I want to take a minute and clear up the confusion about carbohydrates and exercise once and for all. There is absolutely no sense in cutting out carbohydrates; they fuel our bodies.

Our body stores carbohydrates (called "glycogen") in our muscles and our liver. These stored carbohydrates become the primary source of fuel for our brain and muscles after about the first fifteen minutes of a cardio-type exercise. So, if you plan on engaging in any kind of exercise for longer than fifteen minutes and want to feel good doing it, you need to have consumed enough carbohydrates over the past day or two so that your muscles have some glycogen available. If you've ever started a workout and felt like your legs have no power or energy from the get-go, you probably need to eat more carbs such as grains, beans, fruits, and vegetables.

These body boosters are also the brain's preferred source of fuel. When your brain isn't fueled, pretty much everything else in your body suffers. Think of these stores of carbohydrates in your body like canned goods in your pantry. If the power goes out and the food in the fridge goes bad, you turn to those pantry stores. Your body only holds a few hours' worth of stored carbs, and once they've run out, your body will use fat as well as start breaking

THE SAVVY GIRL'S GUIDE TO EXERCISE

EXERCISE IS POSITIVE WHEN . . .

▶ You feel good while doing the activity or workout.

▶ You feel energized after being active.

▶ Your body gains strength and immunity from regular movement.

▶ You feel better mentally and emotionally thanks to the release of dopamine, a feel-good chemical that floods your body during and after physical activity.

▶ You have a clear head because your cells are getting more oxygen from the improved circulation you experience when you move your body.

▶ You feel better throughout a typical day because regular movement makes you feel more agile and comfortable in your body.

EXERCISE IS A PROBLEM WHEN . . .

▶ You're exercising just to control your weight.

▶ You're exercising to give yourself permission to eat.

▶ You get frequent injuries due to overdoing it at the gym.

▶ Your mood suffers because you feel guilty for not working out.

▶ You miss out on adequate sleep in order to exercise, which throws off your hormones, increases cravings, and/or causes you to get sick.

▶ Your life revolves around your workouts to the point of skipping out on fun, social activities.

---

down muscle protein to turn it into a carb-like source of energy. So essentially, not eating enough carbohydrates puts your muscles at risk of weakening and actually prompts your body to hold on to fat.

I know what you're thinking: Why do all of those people on low-carb diets lose weight so fast? The answer: It's the loss of all the canned goods in their body's pantry and the quick breakdown of muscle that happens as a result. For every molecule of glycogen, we also store three molecules of water, so the no-carb eating plan helps people shed water weight quickly. Keep in mind, this is not fat loss. For anyone who exercises, low- and no-carb diets are a great way to slow your metabolism and prompt your body to store fat and lose muscle. This is why monitoring your scale for evidence of progress isn't giving you the full story.

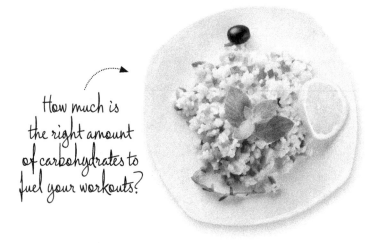

How much is the right amount of carbohydrates to fuel your workouts?

Your old dieting mind wants me to tell you how much to eat. But the truth is, you're going to need a different amount of food every day. The absolute best way to know the right amount of carbohydrates to eat is by eating balanced meals throughout the day and listening to what sounds satisfying. Some days that'll mean you eat a bagel. Other, days you'll have eggs without the toast. Trust what you feel like eating and enjoy those meals without judgment.

THE TRUTH ABOUT CHANGING YOUR BODY

Ready for the cold, hard truth? Not all bodies can get to the same place. So many dieting experts will claim they have the secret to looking like a supermodel, but the truth is that not all women have the ability to look how they think they want to look. This is true no matter how much weight you lose or how many sculpting classes you take. That's why focusing on feeling great in the body you have is a much better way to approach movement.

This may also require some acceptance of what you consider to be your flaws. When it comes to those flaws, know that every single one of us has them. You may or may not have been dealt the proportions and the shape you think you want, but if your goal is happiness, acceptance is the key.

I'm not saying that it's not possible to see changes or results from healthy eating and exercise. However, it's time to make your expectations realistic and take the focus off trying to create a totally different body.

FORGET THE SCALE FOR GOOD
There was a period of time after I became a Savvy Eater when I was working out intensely and quite regularly. I really enjoyed it and loved my newfound strength and endurance. However, after seeing a pretty significant change in the way my body looked, the number on the scale hadn't budged. An increase in muscle and a decrease in fat stores changed my body composition, but I did not lose weight.

Imagine how frustrating that may have felt if I had been looking at the scale for proof that all my effort was paying off. I can guarantee you the old me would have been turned off by the lack of progress on the scale and probably not stuck with the routine that was working—a routine I was also having fun and feeling great doing.

If you decide to focus on the number on the scale or inches lost rather than moving your body in a way that feels good to you, you're almost guaranteed to sabotage yourself. So, put the scale away now. Trust me, you don't need it.

EXERCISE AFFECTS APPETITE

People who exercise vigorously will likely feel some increased hunger. If you enjoy vigorous exercise, by all means, take that high-intensity interval training class. But don't attribute your high hunger to a lack of willpower. Sadly, overexercisers often attribute their body's increased hunger signals to the reason why they have to keep exercising, thus perpetuating a vicious, unhealthy cycle.

GETTING STARTED: YOUR NEW "MOVEMENT" ROUTINE

Creating a movement routine that is right for you starts with ditching the notion of how much you should exercise each week. Also, don't forget that you don't have to sweat to get enough movement. Once you find activities you really love, staying active will feel much more sustainable than trying to hit the gym for an hour or more at a time.

To develop a better relationship with exercise, follow these steps to get savvy about moving:

▶ **REFLECT.** Think about your current workout regimen. Do you dread your workouts or do you love them?

▶ **TAKE A BREAK.** If you aren't fully happy with your exercise routine, consider taking a break and observe how you feel when you don't move your body.

savvy tip Be flexible with what you consider movement. You don't always need to have your running shoes and Lululemon pants on to sneak in some activity. Maybe you start to see windows of opportunity, like a fifteen-minute walk before meeting a friend for lunch or taking the stairs instead of an elevator (small movements add up over time). Do what you can and what you want, and forgive yourself for not always being able to fulfill your plans.

▶**DO WHAT YOU LOVE.** Add more movement into your days when you feel the desire to, but only do what's enjoyable. Also, pay attention to your body during the movement. Do you want to speed up or slow down? Make sure you respond to any pain or discomfort.

▶**REST.** It's crucial to give your body time to recover. Sometimes staying on the couch is what you need and will give you the energy to be active again the next day.

▶**MIX IT UP.** Be conscious of switching up your routine regularly. Your body (and you!) will love the variety.

▶**DON'T TRACK YOURSELF.** Try not to base your movement on how long or how far, or especially how many calories you're burning. See if you can just move for the amount of time that feels right to you. You'll be surprised how great (and freeing) this feels.

Next Up

➔ What you need to know about nutrition

➔ How to avoid the fad diet temptation

➔ Booze: Can you still drink?

Nutrition Truths all Savvy Girls Know

[BRITT: When I decided to become a vegetarian, it wasn't for animal rights or because I was concerned about my karma. All I wanted was a way of eating that would make me healthier (and, let's be honest, skinnier!). At the time, I thought I'd found the Holy Grail, but instead of helping me become healthier, going vegetarian the way I did it backfired. Big-time.

At first, my newfound vegetarianism felt great. I was eating more fruits and vegetables, I had more energy, and I even lost some weight. Friends and colleagues practically cooed when they noticed what a "healthy" eater I was. But it wasn't long until I just couldn't look at another vegetable.

The moment I lost my new-diet beer goggles and got a true glimpse of my diet happened when I was out with friends. The vegetarian choices at most restaurants usually consist of pizza, pasta, or French fries (which, I loved to point out, are usually also vegan). About halfway through dinner one night, I looked over at what my non-vegetarian friend was eating—a chicken-apple-walnut salad—and I remember thinking that her salad looked a lot more satisfying, nourishing, and delicious than my huge bowl of pasta.

In an attempt to be what I thought was healthier, I'd unknowingly steered myself right toward a diet full of refined carbohydrates and low-nutrient foods. By creating an all-or-nothing way of eating, I was actually eating less healthfully. And as we all know by now, the pasta wasn't the problem; it was my "diet rules" (aka my shoulds, can'ts, and don'ts) that were to blame.]

WHAT DOES EATING HEALTHY MEAN?

This can be a tough question to answer when food and nutrition advice is thrown at us from every angle, all the time. As a registered dietitian, I want to help you get nutritionally savvy by knowing some basic, accurate information about how different foods work for our bodies.

But first, a little reminder: As you read this chapter, remind yourself to listen for those old dieting voices telling you what you should eat and what you should not eat. In order to hear what I have to say about nutrition, I need you to check in with yourself and make sure you're not thinking about food as black or white, good or bad—OK?

This also goes for your old shoulds, can'ts, and don'ts. If I encourage you to eat a variety of whole foods, don't hear that and think, "I should eat whole foods, and I am bad if I eat processed foods." If you're saying that to yourself, you missed the point of being a Savvy Eater. Gently pull yourself back to thinking, Satisfaction first, nutrition second. I want to eat to feel good!

One other thing: You don't need to know why a certain food is nutritious or how many vitamins, minerals, and grams of fiber it has to be a healthy eater. All you have to do is eat food and pay attention to how your body feels when and after you eat that food.

WHAT DOES THE "RDN" AFTER SUMNER'S NAME MEAN?
A registered dietitian nutritionist (RDN) is an expert who has achieved a bachelor's degree, followed by completion of a dietetic internship, usually based in a hospital or community clinic, and has passed the national registration exam through the Commission on Dietetic Registration. RDNs also have to achieve continuing-education credits consistently in order to maintain their RDN credential. The simple nutritionist title, on the other hand, has no technical requirements or educational prerequisites, and nutritionists are not held accountable by any association or medical community. Literally anyone who thinks they know about nutrition (whether or not they actually do) can call himself or herself a nutritionist, open an office, advertise, build a website or a blog, or even write a book. Scary, right? So, do your homework if you're getting advice from nutrition "experts." Be a detective and question everything you read and hear, because it may not always be accurate.

THE NUTRITION TRUTHS ALL SAVVY GIRLS KNOW

The Savvy Eater approach to nutrition is centered on understanding that you have permission to eat the foods you want—and when those foods provide a balance of the nutrients your body needs, you'll feel satisfied. That means you're encouraged to throw all of your old diet "rules" out the window. However, there are still some truths about nutrition that can help keep you on your new Savvy Eating track. Here are the most important ones:

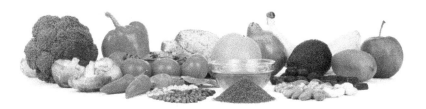

TRUTH NO. 1 ▸ IT'S CRUCIAL TO EAT REAL FOODS

Sounds vague, right? Telling you to eat "real" foods instead of "fake" foods is like me telling you to date a nice guy instead of a jerk. So let me be clear: Real food is food that is closer to its natural form, meaning foods that grow on a tree or come from the ground (think fruits, vegetables, grains, nuts, and legumes as opposed to a bag of potato chips or can of spray cheese).

Of course, not everything you eat is going to be a whole food, and that is fine. Also, I don't want you to get stuck on the number of servings of fruits and vegetables you should have. Instead, keep your fridge stocked with your favorites so they are readily available to add to your meals or have on the side. Eating more real foods will automatically give you more fiber, more vitamins and minerals, and more protective anti-aging antioxidants. I've never had a client tell me they added in more real food and didn't feel better as a result.

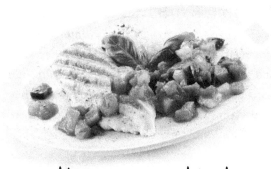

Focus on adding in more real foods to your diet, rather than cutting out foods.

DO YOURSELF A FAVOR AND AVOID TRANS FAT

While Savvy Eating is all about no food being off-limits, it's ideal (when possible) to avoid foods that contain trans fat. Trans fat is a type of fat that gives food a shelf life that's longer than Betty White's career. To steer clear of this ingredient, which is mostly found in packaged foods and commercially baked goods (even seemingly healthy ones, such as protein bars and yogurt-covered raisins!) look for "partially hydrogenated oil" in the ingredients list and "Trans Fat" on the nutrition facts label.

TRUTH NO 2 ▶ HEALTHY EATING IS ALL ABOUT BALANCE

A "balanced" meal means you've got a food (or combo of foods) that gives you carbohydrates, protein, and fat. Our bodies need and use each of these three nutrients for fuel:

▶ **CARBS** keep the metabolism humming, helping you feel consistently energized and alert.

▶ **PROTEIN** triggers satiety hormones and takes longer to break down than carbs, which means it helps you feel fuller longer.

▸ **FAT** helps your body absorb nutrients, provides a "yummy" taste, and, like protein, also takes a while to empty out of your stomach, which contributes to a sense of fullness and satiety.

[BRITT: One of the first diet changes Sumner encouraged me to make was to add protein to my breakfast. Because my first meal of the day lacked protein, I often found myself ravenous by ten a.m. Without the proper nutrition and calories of a balanced meal, all I could focus on was counting down the minutes until it was an "acceptable" lunch hour so I could eat again. Once I started adding a protein at breakfast (eggs, yogurt, turkey, cheese, etc.), everything was completely different. By the time the clock hit noon or even 1:00 p.m., I would calmly think, Oh, I guess I could go grab something for lunch. These days, I almost always try to have a balanced breakfast that includes carbohydrates, fat, and protein.]

The Balance Effect
CARB + PROTEIN + FAT = A BALANCED MEAL

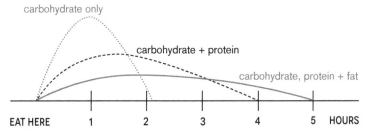

If you eat a high-carbohydrate, low-protein breakfast, insulin levels can increase sharply, causing your blood sugar to crash within 2-2½ hours, stimulating hunger. If you eat a balance of protein, healthy fat, and moderate amounts of carbohydrate, insulin levels will raise more moderately, causing your blood sugar levels and appetite to be at a more even keel.

Source: Reprinted with permission from Susan Dopart, MS, RD, CDE in A Recipe for Life by the Doctor's Dietitian copyright of SGJ Publishing, Inc. 2009

Want easy, balanced meal ideas?
Here are ten:

1. Whole-grain toast (carb) + eggs (protein and fat) + avocado (fat)

2. Apple (carb) + peanut butter (fat and protein) + glass of milk (protein and carb)

3. Rice (carb) + chicken (protein) + veggies cooked in olive oil (fat)

4. Smoothie: Frozen berries and banana (carb) + milk or protein powder (protein) + almond butter or chia seeds (protein and fat)

5. Taco salad: Mixed greens and vegetables + beans and corn (carb) + turkey (protein) + avocado and salad dressing (fat)

6. Salad greens and veggies + grilled fish (protein and fat) + French bread (carb)

7. Pasta and tomato sauce (carb) + ground meat (protein) + broccoli + olive oil and Parmesan cheese (fat)

8. Greek-style yogurt (protein) + walnuts (fat) + chopped fruit and granola (carbs and fat)

9. Oatmeal (carb) + Canadian bacon (protein and fat) + yogurt with fruit and nuts (protein and fat)

10. Tomato soup (carb) + tuna sandwich with cheese (carb, protein, and fat) + carrots

TRUTH NO. 3 ▸ FALLING FOR FAD DIETS IS NEVER A GOOD IDEA

Atkins. Paleo. Diet supplements. Juice detoxes. Anything that promises to be the golden ticket to getting slim is a diet fad to avoid. But, you ask, why is it that my BFF can follow a diet without any of the diet backlash? Well, perhaps it's because that way of eating truly satisfies her, and she doesn't feel deprived or guilty about eating anything off the plan if she wants it. What's right for one person won't necessarily feel right or be right for someone else. First, learn to trust yourself and have peace with food. Then, you can choose to eat or not eat any foods you want.

If you don't like or don't feel good after eating a certain food, avoid it because it doesn't work for your body, not because some diet is telling you to do so.

Here are some of the biggest health trends du jour, plus how to avoid falling prey to the marketing wizards whose job it is to convince you to hop on the bandwagon.

"JUICING" AND DETOX JUICE CLEANSES

Juicing is one of the hottest trends in nutrition these days, yet there's a lot of confusion surrounding the real health pros and cons of juicing. While there's nothing wrong with enjoying a delicious and nutritious veggie and/or fruit juice when you want one, an all-juice "detox" won't help you lose weight for good, get healthier, or detox your body. In fact, your body, when fed well, will detox itself quite well. Your liver and kidneys are working on that 24/7.

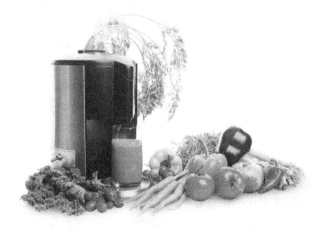

Yes, juice (especially green juice) packs a lot of vitamins, minerals, and antioxidants into one convenient drink. However, juicing also removes the fiber from those fruits and veggies and concentrates the sugars, which can spike your blood-sugar level. Juice also lacks the triple-threat combo (carbs, protein, and fat), meaning it's a pretty poor meal substitute.

So, go ahead and order that $9 organic, cold-pressed, kale-celery-ginger juice if you're craving one—just sip it as part of a balanced diet rather than thinking it's your ticket to perfect health.

PALEO, ATKINS, AND THE LOW- AND NO-CARB CRAZE

Every time I see a new client who is afraid to eat carbs and has tried the no-/low-carb way of eating, her story goes something like this: "I cut carbs, lost ten pounds, started eating carbs again, gained all of the weight back, and now I'm afraid to eat carbs. Oh, and when I start eating them, I can't stop."

Sound familiar?

Here's the deal: When you stop eating carbohydrates, your body uses up all of its stored carbs. When those stored carbs are gone, you lose some water weight as a result. So, the number on the scale goes down, you feel lighter, and you think, I can do this! I'm being good and getting results! And then you meet a bagel you simply cannot resist. And a piece of pizza. And a bowl of penne à la vodka. Soon, you're overeating carbs and the weight comes back on. (Water weight comes back about as fast as wetting a dried-out sponge.) Even worse, you're attributing that weight gain to adding back carbs, when really it's a result of the overeating you are doing as a consequence of depriving yourself when you were on the low- or no-carb diet.

THE NO-SUGAR PHENOMENON

How many times have you heard a trendy friend talk about her new, sugar-free diet? Well, my Savvy Eaters, here is what you need to know about sugar so you can nod politely—then have your cake and eat it too.

Many of us are eating too much sugar these days. Nobody can argue with that fact. However, cutting all sugar from your diet for the long haul is completely unrealistic. It would mean birthdays with no birthday cake, Thanksgiving with no pumpkin pie, Christmas with no sugar cookies . . . you get my drift.

The truth is, if you can stop feeling bad about eating sugar, you can stop being ashamed for wanting it. It's that simple, really! Eat a cookie, stay present, and ask yourself with each bite...

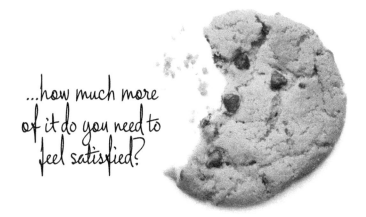

...how much more of it do you need to feel satisfied?

TRUTH NO. 4 ▸ DRINK THE SAME WAY YOU EAT—MINDFULLY

Swirl, sniff, sip . . . there's nothing quite like a lovely glass of vino to help take away the stress of the day, right? Or that extra-large iced coffee to get you going in the morning (or keep you going in the middle of the afternoon)? There is no problem with having a drink or enjoying that caffeine hit when you really want it. Yet if you're habitually using alcohol, coffee, or another beverage to unwind, perk up at work, improve your mood, or escape your feelings, it's time to get savvy about what you drink.

While I'm not telling you to be a total teetotaler or water warrior, I am encouraging you to be aware of how much you consume. What is your body telling you if you have an energy crash or feel jittery from too much soda or coffee? Are you feeling uncomfortable about the unintentional weight gain you've noticed since you started having soda or wine with meals?

If you find that you turn to these sugary or alcoholic beverages out of habit, focus on paying attention to how they make you feel, just like you're practicing with the food you eat. And remember, just as with emotional eating, it's important for your health to get real about mindless or automatic drinking.

Next Up

➔ How long will it take to become a Savvy Eater?

➔ What challenges you'll face along the way

➔ How to get back on track if you find yourself slipping into old habits

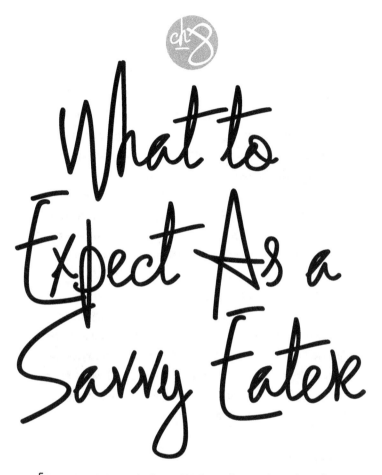

What to Expect As a Savvy Eater

[**BRITT**: I wish I could tell you that I was Sumner's perfect client and that I sailed through this process. Nope. Instead I was more like the kid in class who gets easily distracted.

Although I did notice immediate changes, such as how good it felt to ditch feeling guilty if I ate anything that wasn't a vegetable and how freeing it felt not to worry about every last bite of food I consumed, the real change—making Savvy Eating feel completely natural—took several months. Mostly because (a) I had tried to diet again (fine, two times) and (b) I got hung up on the no-forbidden-foods thing and unknowingly attributed eating healthy to "dieting" even if I actually wanted to eat healthy.

It was hard for me not to get lured in by new diets and gizmos. It was all my friends seemed to want to talk about at dinner and I'd wonder if I'd get left behind if I didn't participate. For example, one spring my friend flashed her new activity tracker at me during brunch. It looked so cool and high-tech. It could track her sleep, her calorie intake, and her activity level. "I've already lost four pounds," she said. Distracted by her shiny new toy and how it was almost bikini season, I just couldn't help myself. After brunch I stopped by a big-box electronics store and got myself my own shiny gizmo. "It can't hurt to try it!" I said to myself in hopes of justifying my departure from not-dieting.

But like Sumner predicted, that little toy began to annoy the crap out of me. Some days I needed more food than was "allowed" in my calorie budget and the bright-red message that read you're over your budget (aka "failure alert") was making me feel bad about myself. Not to mention the pedometer . . . beeping at me to get my daily 10,000 steps (which, by the way, is a lot of steps). One day the tracker ended up in the washing machine and I was relieved when it didn't turn on again.

I also remember when Sumner had to remind me that it was OK to eat healthy, and that making healthy choices didn't make me a dieter. I was so hung up on making sure I didn't judge myself for my food choices and that no foods were off limits that I forgot to ask myself if I actually wanted the turkey burger and fries. Just because you can eat the greasiest thing on the menu, that doesn't mean you need to order it. It's about giving yourself permission to eat what you want, and if you want to order a salad because you're craving something fresh and healthy, that is being a Savvy Eater.

My ups and downs—as well as some other ones you may experience—are what this chapter is all about. The more you understand what to expect during your Savvy Eating transition and know which common roadblocks could threaten to set you back, the less likely you'll be to throw in the towel before everything finally clicks. And it will click. Trust me.]

While we all want change right now, it's important to realize that once you master the concepts of being a Savvy Eater, you will be set for life. For some, the transition is fairly quick. It might take a few weeks to a couple of months. However for most, it can be several months or years! Yes, I said it: years. But don't interpret that as a bad thing. Even if it takes what seems like forever to master being a Savvy Eater, you will still see benefits and many positive changes immediately.

Learning to be a Savvy Eater is kind of like learning a new language. If you consistently practice the language, it becomes easier and easier, no matter how long it takes to become fluent. When you look at it that way, it's easier to be patient when the non-dieting way of eating isn't happening as fast as you think it should. The same way a student learning French will eventually dream in French, Savvy Eaters will eventually catch themselves eating as a Savvy Eater without even thinking about it. And when that happens, you won't imagine ever going back to the yo-yo emotions of dieting.

THE FIVE SAVVY EATING PHASES YOU'LL EXPERIENCE

There are a few phases you will go through when transitioning from a dieter to a Savvy Eater—and it helps to be aware of these so you know what you're dealing with when it inevitably pops up for you:

PHASE 1 ▶ DIET ROCK BOTTOM

This is where you land right before you're ready to kiss dieting good-bye. It's what drew you to this book in the first place. It's at Diet Rock Bottom when you realize you're ready to stop dieting because it simply doesn't work. You're ready to find a way to not feel bad all the time about your body and your eating. You're absolutely convinced all the money, time, intense workouts, and emotional energy you've spent dieting hasn't gotten you anywhere.

PHASE 2 ▶ PERMISSION TO EAT (AKA THE HONEYMOON PHASE)

Here's when you throw out your "bad foods" list and work toward breaking up with Guilt and Shame. You start to give yourself permission to eat what you really want for the first time in a long time. This stage is exciting, freeing, and fun because you get to rediscover what satiety really means and what it feels like to enjoy your food without feeling bad. I often refer to this as the Honeymoon Phase because clients can't believe how well it works and it can feel too good to be true. They're amazed that they did not eat everything in sight.

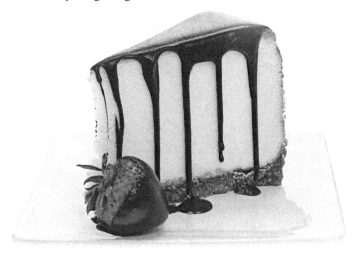

PHASE 3 ▸ LEARNING TO KNOW WHEN IT'S NOT FOOD YOU NEED

After taking away the deprivation, you can focus on why you're eating—this part is the key to limiting and eventually putting an end to emotional eating. By learning to know when it's not food you need, without being clouded by deprivation and rebellion, you are better able to cut down on eating excess food. Yes, weight normalization can happen when you make this shift if you're not currently at the right weight for your body.

PHASE 4 ▸ BUILDING TRUST WITH YOURSELF

This transition to trusting yourself around food happens after eating a variety of foods and discovering that some make you feel great while others sap your energy, make you feel bloated, or give you a stomachache. When you stop judging yourself for your food choices and trust your intuition, you realize you no longer need food rules.

PHASE 5 ▸ MASTERING SAVVY EATING AND A POSITIVE BODY IMAGE

During this stage, you're much calmer around food and not so worried all the time. You frequently finish meals feeling comfortable and satisfied. However, it's also very normal if you still notice old dieting thoughts or negative voices creeping into your mind from time to time. You may still struggle with body image, although not nearly on the level that you used to.

This is also the phase where you'll notice that you enjoy eating more healthful foods, because although you have permission to eat whatever you want, you realize that eating more real, wholesome and good-for-you grub ultimately makes you feel your best.

This is the phase when I remind my clients that it's OK to eat healthfully. Just because you want to eat natural, nutritious foods, that does not mean you are dieting.

SEVEN ROAD BLOCKS YOU MIGHT FACE

While going through the five phases above, many barriers can pop up that might make you question your newfound freedom to eat. Everyone, and I mean everyone, experiences road blocks during the transition to eating intuitively. It's normal. It's part of the process. It's a sign that you're learning.

So, when you find yourself struggling with a part of the process, tell yourself, This doesn't mean I'm failing or that I can't be a Savvy Eater; it just means I'm still learning.

Here are some common road blocks you may face and how to move past them:

ROAD BLOCK NO. 1 ▶ YOU'RE STILL LOOKING FOR A DIET

If you catch yourself doing this, it means you're still judging yourself and your food choices, probably because you don't really believe you have permission to eat what you want.

THE FIX ▶ Remind yourself over and over again that the dieting cycle is no fun, hasn't gotten you anywhere, and is a short-term process that always ends in failure. Savvy Eating is a way of eating that takes time to master but will work for the rest of your life. Isn't that worth putting the effort into?

[BRITT: Don't be surprised if you end up back here again even though you've read this book and have had a few successful months not dieting. As you already know, after a few appointments with Sumner, I attempted to diet again—and it put me right back into the unpleasant dieting cycle, meaning I eventually hit Dieting Rock Bottom all over again. I called Sumner (she wasn't surprised), booked another session, and finally decided to give the non-dieting approach 100 percent effort and commitment. You know what they say: If at first you don't succeed: try, try again. And also: misery loves company. So if you get here again, remember I did too. You're not alone.]

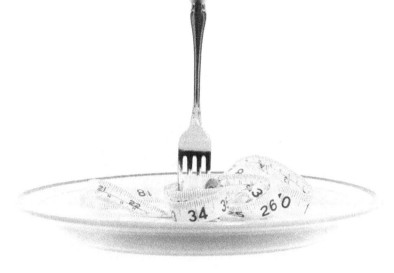

What you should take away from Brittany's story is that many of you will still try to diet again, and that is part of breaking the habit. Sometimes we need a reminder of what doesn't work to help us learn what does. When you feel yourself falling into the dieting cycle again, remember this story and come back to this book, because you deserve to eat in a way that feels good for you.

ROAD BLOCK NO. 2 ▸ YOU'RE GIVING YOURSELF PSEUDO-PERMISSION

Giving yourself full permission to eat is harder than it sounds, which is why this is such an expected road block. Look at what you've been told both directly and subliminally for years: As a woman, you're supposed to watch what you eat, weigh less, and rid your body of all unnecessary fat, right? Wrong! As you're learning to give yourself full permission, it also doesn't help to be constantly bombarded with dieting-mentality messages in blogs, magazines, books, and ads that tempt you to go back to believing that you can't trust yourself or that healthy eating is all or nothing.

THE FIX ▸ Try granting yourself full permission to eat anything your heart desires for just one week. Once time is up, reassess and determine how that felt. If you ate and felt out of control, realize that it is due to all of the built-up deprivation—not because you gave yourself permission. There's a good chance you'll be surprised that it took less food than you expected to feel satisfied.

ONE MEAL WON'T CHANGE YOUR BODY

Remember that there is no one food or one meal that makes you gain weight. Weight gain typically happens as a result of eating more food than your body needs over a period of time and eating for reasons other than hunger. Refocus your efforts on being mindful (listen for those cues on when to eat, what you're craving, and when to stop), instead of on "good" foods and "bad" foods.

ROAD BLOCK NO. 3 ▸ YOUR FRIENDS AND/OR FAMILY ARE CONSTANTLY DISCUSSING THE RECENT SUCCESS OF THEIR SUPER-RESTRICTIVE DIET

This is something you may not be able to escape, and it's natural to feel uncomfortable in these types of conversations as you learn to be a Savvy Eater.

THE FIX ▸ Remind yourself that people love to brag about their diets, but no one brags about how hard it is to maintain a restrictive diet, the secret eating, the obsessing over food, and the inevitable weight gain when they reintroduce the formerly forbidden foods back into their diet. Make an agreement with yourself that you don't need to participate in these diet conversations and that other people can do whatever they want. Your friend can go ahead and try that super-restrictive diet—but you'll go ahead and pass if she tries to make you her diet buddy.

ROAD BLOCK NO. 4 ▸ YOU'RE STILL EMOTIONALLY EATING

Addressing your emotional needs takes a lot of practice and a lot of forgiveness, but you'll notice that as time passes, small changes are taking place and building on one another. When I'm agitated, anxious, or bored, the old emotional eater in me still starts looking for something to eat to deal with how I'm feeling. The difference now is that I have strengthened the skill of being present, and I'm better able to recognize that eating for emotional reasons is a choice.

THE FIX ▸ You just need more practice. Remind yourself that eating for emotional reasons does not make you a failure or a bad person, and quit beating yourself up about it. No one meal or experience changes your body, so learn from it, move on, and know that change comes from having compassion for yourself for what you were going through. Also, don't be afraid to ask for help if you're eating because of depression or you're going through stressful life situations. Getting support with the things that are bugging you is the fastest and most productive way to get to the bottom of your feelings and the key to making positive changes for good.

ROAD BLOCK NO. 5 ▸ YOU'RE STUCK FOCUSING ON WEIGHT LOSS

If you're still trying to reduce the number on the scale, you're stuck in the dieting cycle, which is the root of your eating issues. What we know about dieting is that it is the number-one predictor of weight gain. Your body weight is not something you can entirely control. Genetics and metabolism are responsible for your weight as well. We are not all designed to be the same weight.

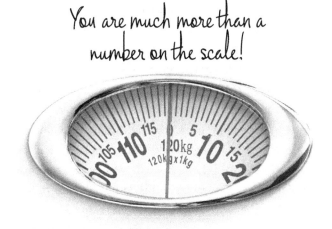

You are much more than a number on the scale!

THE FIX ▶ What can you look at other than weight loss for reassurance that this is the right way of eating for you? Have you stopped bingeing? Have you stopped beating yourself up after eating? Are you enjoying food more and worrying about food less? Do you feel better after eating because you stop at the right point? See, you don't need a scale to know if this new way of eating is working. If your body does have weight to lose, then it's likely that weight change will happen gradually—not within a few short weeks. You may also need to work on being patient and learning to love your body no matter what your weight. The more you love and accept yourself, the better self-care you will be willing to practice, and that is how you'll ultimately be your healthiest.

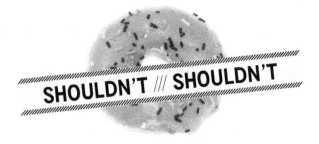

SHOULDN'T /// SHOULDN'T

ROAD BLOCK NO. 6: YOU'RE STILL HEARING SHOULDS

You might notice you're still trying to find out what you should be eating or when you should stop eating. Judging yourself in this way will stall or slow your Savvy Eating progress.

THE FIX ▶ Start by replacing all the shoulds with questions about what you feel and need. For example, if someone offers you dessert after dinner and you automatically think, I shouldn't have all of this, replace that thought with, Where am I on the Hunger and Fullness Spectrum? If I eat this, will I still be at a comfortable level of fullness? And how much of this do I need to eat to feel satisfied? Remember, if you think you should stop sooner than you really want to, you're setting yourself up for rebellious eating.

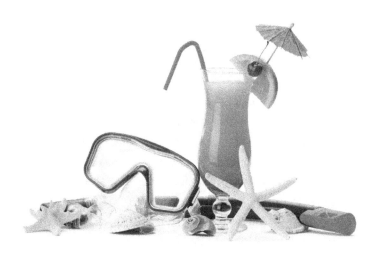

ROAD BLOCK NO. 7: YOU STRUGGLE WHEN EATING AT SPECIAL EVENTS OR ON VACATION

When you're home and in your routine, being a Savvy Eater works. However, at a special event or on vacation, you find it easy to overeat.

THE FIX ▶ Spend five to ten minutes alone before the event or vacation and visualize how you expect your eating to go. Picture yourself staying calm around food and continuing to offer yourself total permission to eat what you want. Remind yourself to stay mindful of how much you need to feel comfortably full and satisfied.

Expect to work a little harder at changing your approach to eating in these situations. For many years, these were your chances to indulge and cheat on your diet! Forgive yourself for all the past overeating or restricting you've done at similar events and recognize that the fears you may have about your eating are legitimate.

Then, trust that you now have more tools and information to make this time different. Don't expect perfection (whatever that would mean), but expect yourself to stay connected to what your body is telling you.

Ready to be on your way? ...

No matter what road blocks you've faced or where you find yourself today, I want you to know that Savvy Eating is within your reach. You are ready to move forward from the discontent of dieting to feeling amazing in your body—for good.

This book was written for the authentic intuitive eater in you who knows exactly what she wants and needs, and you've already taken the first step toward rediscovering her. You're done with restriction and deprivation. You're done constantly feeling guilty. And you're done eating just to escape something else. You know as much as I do that you deserve so much more. You now have everything you need to get going. You're officially on your way to the rest of your diet-free life.

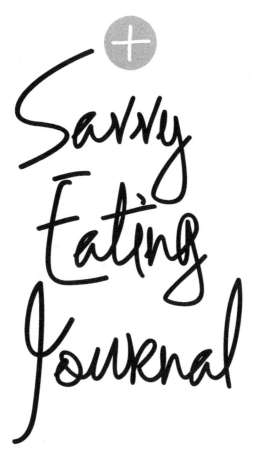

Savvy Eating Journal

Start getting savvy with this Savvy Eating journal!

Simply record the time of day, your hunger level before eating, your location, and short notes on your mood, what you ate, and your level of fullness after eating. An example has been filled in for you as a guideline. Also be sure to tune in to your satisfaction. Remember, being a Savvy Eater is about listening to your body, and eating to feel satisfied. This journal is designed to be a tool for you to help adjust away from an old automatic eating behavior toward a more mindful, connected way of eating. Don't let yourself get caught up in judging what you record; simply use it as a way to be more mindful.

TIME	LEVEL OF HUNGER High Medium Low	LOCATION / MOOD NOTES	WHAT I ATE	LEVEL OF FULLNESS High Medium Low	AM I SATISFIED? Yes / No
7:00 am	H (M) L	Home / Tired	Yogurt and cereal	H (M) L	(Y) / N
	H M L			H M L	Y / N
	H M L			H M L	Y / N
	H M L			H M L	Y / N
	H M L			H M L	Y / N
	H M L			H M L	Y / N
	H M L			H M L	Y / N
	H M L			H M L	Y / N
	H M L			H M L	Y / N
	H M L			H M L	Y / N
	H M L			H M L	Y / N
	H M L			H M L	Y / N

TIME	LEVEL OF HUNGER High Medium Low	LOCATION / MOOD NOTES	WHAT I ATE	LEVEL OF FULLNESS High Medium Low	AM I SATISFIED? Yes / No
	H M L			H M L	Y / N
	H M L			H M L	Y / N
	H M L			H M L	Y / N
	H M L			H M L	Y / N
	H M L			H M L	Y / N
	H M L			H M L	Y / N
	H M L			H M L	Y / N
	H M L			H M L	Y / N
	H M L			H M L	Y / N
	H M L			H M L	Y / N
	H M L			H M L	Y / N
	H M L			H M L	Y / N

TIME	LEVEL OF HUNGER High Medium Low	LOCATION / MOOD NOTES	WHAT I ATE	LEVEL OF FULLNESS High Medium Low	AM I SATISFIED? Yes / No
	H M L			H M L	Y / N
	H M L			H M L	Y / N
	H M L			H M L	Y / N
	H M L			H M L	Y / N
	H M L			H M L	Y / N
	H M L			H M L	Y / N
	H M L			H M L	Y / N
	H M L			H M L	Y / N
	H M L			H M L	Y / N
	H M L			H M L	Y / N
	H M L			H M L	Y / N
	H M L			H M L	Y / N

TIME	LEVEL OF HUNGER High Medium Low	LOCATION / MOOD NOTES	WHAT I ATE	LEVEL OF FULLNESS High Medium Low	AM I SATISFIED? Yes / No
	H M L			H M L	Y / N
	H M L			H M L	Y / N
	H M L			H M L	Y / N
	H M L			H M L	Y / N
	H M L			H M L	Y / N
	H M L			H M L	Y / N
	H M L			H M L	Y / N
	H M L			H M L	Y / N
	H M L			H M L	Y / N
	H M L			H M L	Y / N
	H M L			H M L	Y / N
	H M L			H M L	Y / N

TIME	LEVEL OF HUNGER High Medium Low	LOCATION / MOOD NOTES	WHAT I ATE	LEVEL OF FULLNESS High Medium Low	AM I SATISFIED? Yes / No
	H M L			H M L	Y / N
	H M L			H M L	Y / N
	H M L			H M L	Y / N
	H M L			H M L	Y / N
	H M L			H M L	Y / N
	H M L			H M L	Y / N
	H M L			H M L	Y / N
	H M L			H M L	Y / N
	H M L			H M L	Y / N
	H M L			H M L	Y / N
	H M L			H M L	Y / N
	H M L			H M L	Y / N

TIME	LEVEL OF HUNGER High Medium Low	LOCATION / MOOD NOTES	WHAT I ATE	LEVEL OF FULLNESS High Medium Low	AM I SATISFIED? Yes / No
	H M L			H M L	Y / N
	H M L			H M L	Y / N
	H M L			H M L	Y / N
	H M L			H M L	Y / N
	H M L			H M L	Y / N
	H M L			H M L	Y / N
	H M L			H M L	Y / N
	H M L			H M L	Y / N
	H M L			H M L	Y / N
	H M L			H M L	Y / N
	H M L			H M L	Y / N
	H M L			H M L	Y / N

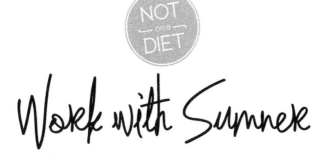

Work with Sumner

NEED MORE SUPPORT? Want to talk through your unique experiences and struggles and get personalized advice to help take you from dieter to Savvy Eater? You have the option to work one-on-one with Sumner or someone on her team to help you make the changes we've described in this book. If you struggle with chronic dieting, binge eating, or an eating disorder such as anorexia or bulimia, please reach out for help.

Sumner is available to work with you in person or via web video or phone sessions to help you get to the bottom of your eating struggles and find peace with food and your body once and for all. To inquire about setting up a private session, call 800-675-3193 or send an e-mail to info@NotOnADiet.com and mention "Savvy Eating" for a special offer of 20 percent off your first month of sessions.

HAVE EATING QUESTIONS? Tweet your Q's to Sumner at @ MyDietitian. Follow along with Not on a Diet on Facebook for motivation, meal inspiration, and reminders that you don't need to diet to be healthy and happy.

Acknowledgments

This book would not have been possible without the dedication, hard work, creativity, and patience of the following people:

Content Editor: **MEGHAN RABBITT**

Copyeditor: **RACHELLE MANDIK**

Cover and Interior Designer: **TARA LONG**

BRITTANY'S ACKNOWLEDGMENTS

A SPECIAL THANKS . . .

TO MEGHAN ▶ Yep. Definitely won the Lotto! Not only are you an amazing editor, but you're also a dream to work with. Thanks for always being honest with your feedback and for taking a high level of care with these books. I'm looking forward to working with you on many more projects!

TO SUMNER ▶ Being able to enjoy food and be free from guilt and shame is one of the best gifts I have ever been given. You are so passionate about what you do, and that shines through in everything you do. It was an honor to do this collaboration with you. Thanks for helping all of us Savvy Girls get free from dieting.

TO TARA ▶ You have such an eye for design and you continue to blow away my expectations. Thanks for making the design of the Savvy Girl books better than I could have imagined. I am so grateful to have you a part of the Savvy Girl team!

TO RACHELLE ▶ Thanks for taking a high level of care with these Savvy Girl books and for going above and beyond! I am so happy to have you as part of the Savvy Girl team.

TO LOU: ▶ To think that only four years ago I told you about my crazy idea for a book series while we were in the middle of the Bolivian Amazon. You believed in me from the start and your support has never wavered. You are my rock, my best friend, and the love of my life.

TO MY PARENTS ▶ I am so lucky to have parents that instilled in me a love for adventure and a strong work ethic. Without both there would be no Savvy Girl. Thank you for all of your love, support, and guidance as I go after my dream. I love you both more than anything.

TO MY BROTHER ▶ I couldn't ask for a better brother. I feel so lucky that we have become so close and that we get to hang out all the time. It makes my heart melt that you always carry a copy of my Savvy Girl books in your briefcase. Your support means the world to me.

TO SEAN ▶ Thank you for believing in me from the beginning and for making sure I kept myself a part of the books instead of hiding behind the scenes as I had originally planned. I have you to thank for this pivotal detail in the progression of Savvy Girl.

TO MY GIRLFRIENDS ▶ I couldn't do this without all of the love and support from you all! Love you girls!

ADDITIONAL THANK-YOUS ▶ Thank you to Diana for also contributing on the editing side of this book. I am thrilled to have you a part of the Savvy Girl team.

SUMNER'S ACKNOWLEDGMENTS

A SPECIAL THANKS...

TO MY DAUGHTER ▶ You were with me every day, growing in my belly for the nine months we worked on this book. You have been my ultimate inspiration to share this information with girls and women everywhere, so that we can create a culture of self-love and peace with eating, and open ourselves to all the possibilities life has to offer. You are my love.

TO MY CLIENTS ▶ I wouldn't be able to do what I love to do for a living without you. Each of your stories has reinforced to me the power we all have to change what isn't working and that it is possible for women to love and respect their natural bodies even in a culture that tries to convince us otherwise.

TO JOHNNY ▶ Thank you for letting me bounce my thoughts off of you during many late evenings when I knew you were already drained from the day. Thank you for being excited with me when I needed it. Your support, patience, and never-ending encouragement for me to forge my own path and be a maverick in this field means more than you'll ever know. You bring me up when I'm down. You're the best.

TO MY MENTOR AND TEACHER, ELYSE ▶ Without your guidance, I would never have found all that Intuitive Eating has to offer. Your wisdom has become such a special part of my life and the lives of so many who have come to me. I'm forever thankful.

A Note from Brittany

Thanks for reading! Now get back to that fabulous life! ;)

XO
Brittany

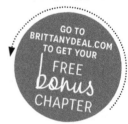

GO TO BRITTANYDEAL.COM TO GET YOUR FREE *bonus* CHAPTER

OTHER SAVVY GIRL GUIDEBOOKS:

Savvy Girl, A Guide to Wine by Brittany Deal

Savvy Girl, A Guide to Etiquette by Brittany Deal and Bren Underwood

Join the community at BrittanyDeal.com to be notified when the next Savvy Girl guidebook is published. Or follow me on social media to stay in the loop.

THE PURSUIT OF SAVVY:

Check out my blog "The Pursuit of Savvy" on BrittanyDeal.com and join me in the pursuit to get savvy and get the most out of life!

INTERESTED IN COLLABORATING WITH SAVVY GIRL?

Are you an expert on a topic? E-mail me at hello@savvygirl.net or contact me via social media about collaborating on a Savvy Girl guidebook or on articles at BrittanyDeal.com.

CPSIA information can be obtained
at www.ICGtesting.com
Printed in the USA
BVHW080515291119
565150BV00007B/282/P

9 780989 710978